Heart Teams for Treatment of Cardiovascular Disease

Thierry Mesana
Editor

Heart Teams for Treatment of Cardiovascular Disease

A Guide for Advancing Patient-Centered Cardiac Care

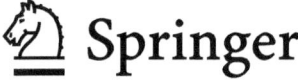 Springer

Editor
Thierry Mesana
University of Ottawa Heart Institute
Ottawa, ON
Canada

ISBN 978-3-030-19123-8   ISBN 978-3-030-19124-5   (eBook)
https://doi.org/10.1007/978-3-030-19124-5

This Springer imprint is published by the registered company Springer Nature Switzerland AG
The registered company address is: Gewerbestrasse 11, 6330 Cham, Switzerland

"Coming together is a beginning, staying together is progress, working together is success"
Henry Ford (July 30, 1863–April 7, 1947)
Founder of the Ford Motor Company

"It is amazing what you can accomplish if you do not care who gets the credit"
Harry S. **Truman** (May 8, 1884–December 26, 1972)
33rd President of the United States (1945–1953)

Foreword

Cardiovascular care often requires the involvement of multiple subspecialties to deliver state-of-the-art care to the patients. The classic model of care is based on silos where patients are being assessed and referred to the next point of treatment with no true multidisciplinary discussion. The growing clinical complexity in patient acuity, the aging population, and the new and expensive technologies necessitate a change in the way we make clinical decisions about patients. We need an integrated and evidence-based approach across disciplines to replace the classic care model.

The introduction of catheter-based valve technologies provides an excellent platform in providing care to cardiovascular patients using the Heart Team concept. This concept is very well suited to support a patient-centered approach in which the decision-making process is supported by a multidisciplinary team. This Heart Team approach is no longer unique to structural heart disease as in many centers multidisciplinary discussions take place around coronary artery disease, arrhythmia, and heart failure. The Heart Team can further advance the care of the patient by sharing and discussing local institutional data that is related to a specific disease process, be it coronary artery disease, structural heart disease, arrhythmia, or heart failure, and tailor the best treatment option to patients within the same institution. The University of Ottawa Heart Institute has been leading the expansion of the Heart Team concept for years now, and the pioneering work done by Dr. Thierry Mesana as the leader of the organization with his colleagues is remarkable.

This textbook contains up-to-date information on the current state of the Heart Team concept across different clinical situations and disciplines, or even original themes such as the Women's Heart Health. The readers can find invaluable information on the function of the heart team, decision-making process, and improved delivery of care from very experienced physicians, some of whom pioneered the model and experienced firsthand its evolution. The information in the book provides effective tools and references designed to enhance knowledge and understanding of the workflow. In this ever-changing and more complex clinical world, this book provides a roadmap for the journey ahead.

College Park, MD, USA   Niv Ad

Preface

T.E.A.M (Together, Everyone Achieves More)

The concept of Heart Team is associated with a multidisciplinary approach involving an inter-professional group of cardiovascular medical experts working together. With the development of new technologies, such as catheter-based valve therapies, together with the increasing complexities of cardiovascular patients, Heart Teams have set a new standard of care and represent a significant marker of high quality of care.

This book is first of its kind as far as the related subject matter, and it is meant to reach out to all healthcare professionals—including all caregivers beyond physicians and administrators—who believe that teamwork is the very first element of excellence in patient care.

You will find a variety of chapters that can help healthcare organizations and medical leaders starting or expanding Heart Teams in different areas. We do not believe that there is a singular model for Heart Team development. Heart Teams more commonly address disease-specific issues and questions, such as valve disease, coronary artery disease, or cardiac arrhythmias. For instance, how do we overcome logistical or cultural challenges to successfully build Heart Teams in coronary artery disease? How can valve specialists best work together? This book does not provide magic solutions to these challenges. Instead, it engages physicians and co-workers to think out of the box, building a team model adapted to their environment.

This book also describes how Heart Teams can be beneficial to address specific issues in critical areas such as cardiac intensive care or cardiac imaging. A team approach is quite relevant in such high-resource intensity areas in order to achieve high-quality and cost-efficient care. How do we make sure that the right patient has the right test at the right moment? Are patients in cardiology critical care units so different than postoperative surgical patients? How to integrate cardiologists, surgeons, and critical care specialists in a new model of intensive care unit?

I would like to give my most sincere gratitude to each contributing author of each chapter in this book and thank them for sharing their experience and vision. This was a hard work and great teamwork!

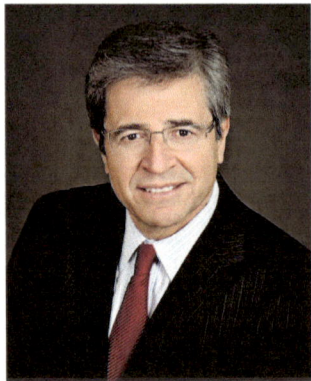

Ottawa, ON, Canada   Thierry Mesana

Contents

Contributors

Mark Ainslie, MBChB, MRCP, PhD, CCDS, CCEP-A Lancashire Cardiac Centre, Department of Cardiac Electrophysiology, Blackpool, UK

Talal Al-Atassi, MD, CM, MPH, FRCSC University of Ottawa Heart Institute, Department of Surgery, Division of Cardiac Surgery, Ottawa, ON, Canada

Rob Beanlands, MD, FRCPC, FACC, FCCS Division of Cardiology, University of Ottawa Heart Institute, Ottawa, ON, Canada

David Hugh Birnie, BSc, MB ChB, MRCP, MD Division of Cardiology, University of Ottawa Heart Institute, Ottawa, ON, Canada

Jacinthe Boulet, MDCM, BsC McGill University Health Centre, Department of Cardiology, Montreal, QC, Canada

Renzo Cecere, MD, FRCSC McGill University Health Centre, Department of Cardiology, Montreal, QC, Canada

Vincent Chan, MD, MPH Department of Surgery, University of Ottawa Heart Institute, Ottawa, ON, Canada

Aun-Yeong Chong, BSc, MBBS, MRCP, MD University of Ottawa Heart Institute, Department of Cardiology, Ottawa, ON, Canada

Benjamin J. W. Chow, MD Division of Cardiology, University of Ottawa Heart Institute, Ottawa, ON, Canada

Thais Coutinho, MD University of Ottawa Heart Institute, Department of Cardiology, Ottawa, ON, Canada

Andrew Michael Crean, MRCP, FRCR, MPhil, FSCMR, MPH Division of Cardiology, University of Ottawa Heart Institute, Ottawa, ON, Canada

Nadia Giannetti, MD, FRCPC McGill University Health Centre, Department of Cardiology, Montreal, QC, Canada

David Glineur, MD, PhD Cardiac Surgery, University of Ottawa Heart Institute, Ottawa, ON, Canada

Benjamin Hibbert, MD, PhD Department of Medicine, Division of Cardiology, University of Ottawa Heart Institute, Ottawa, ON, Canada

Alison M. Hosey University of Ottawa Heart Institute, Research Services, Ottawa, ON, Canada

Daniel Juneau, MD Centre Hospitalier de l'Université de Montréal (CHUM), Department of Nuclear Medicine, Montreal, QC, Canada

Division of Cardiology, University of Ottawa Heart Institute, Ottawa, ON, Canada

Marino Labinaz, MD, FRCPC, FACC University of Ottawa Heart Institute, Division of Cardiology, Ottawa, ON, Canada

Krystina B. Lewis, RN, MN, PhD, CCN(C) University of Ottawa School of Nursing, Ottawa, ON, Canada

Peter P. Liu University of Ottawa Heart Institute, Departments of Medicine/ Cellular and Molecular Medicine, Ottawa, ON, Canada

Terry Meadows University of Ottawa Heart Institute, Ottawa, ON, Canada

Thierry Mesana, MD, PhD University of Ottawa Heart Institute, Ottawa, ON, Canada

David Messika-Zeitoun, MD, PhD Division of Cardiology, University of Ottawa Heart Institute, Ottawa, ON, Canada

Jennifer L. Reed, BPHE, BA, MEd CS, PhD University of Ottawa Heart Institute, Department of Exercise Physiology and Cardiovascular Health Lab, Division of Cardiac Prevention and Rehabilitation, Ottawa, ON, Canada

Norvinda Rodger, B.Comm, MPH Department of Clinical Services, University of Ottawa Heart Institute, Ottawa, ON, Canada

Heather Sherrard, BscN, MHA, CHE Department of Clinical Services, University of Ottawa Heart Institute, Ottawa, ON, Canada

Anthony Tran, MD, MS University of Connecticut Health, Department of Surgery, Farmington, CT, USA

Abbreviations

AAA	Abdominal aortic aneurysms
ACC	American College of Cardiology
ACHD	Adult congenital heart disease
AF	Atrial fibrillation
AHA	American Heart Association
ARB	Angiotensin receptor blocker
ARNi	Angiotensin receptor neprilysin inhibitor
AS	Aortic valve stenosis
ASCEND-HF	Acute Study of Clinical Effectiveness of Nesiritide and Decompensated Heart Failure
AUC	Appropriate use criteria
AV	Atrioventricular [node]
CABG	Coronary artery bypass graft
CAD	Coronary artery disease
CCU	Coronary care unit
CEO	Chief executive officer
CHD	Coronary heart disease
CI	Confidence interval
CICU	Coronary Intensive Care Unit
CIED(s)	Cardiac implantable electronic device(s)
CMAJ	*Canadian Medical Association Journal*
CMR	Cardiac magnetic resonance
CR	Cardiac rehabilitation
CRT	Cardiac resynchronization therapy
CSICU	Cardiac Surgical Intensive Care Unit
CT	Computed tomography
CVICU	Cardiovascular intensive care unit
DECIDE	Decision-making and choices to inform dialogue and empower AF patients [Center]
ECMO	Extracorporeal membrane oxygenation
EEV	Encircling endocardial ventriculotomy
EHRA	European Heart Rhythm Association
EMR	Electronic medical record
ER	Endocardial resection

ESC	European Society of Cardiology
HEART	Heart Failure Etiology and Analysis Research Team
HT	Heart team
ICU	Intensive care unit
JAMA	*Journal of the American Medical Association*
JACC	*Journal of the American College of Cardiology*
ICD(s)	Implantable cardioverter defibrillator(s)
IHD	Ischemic heart disease
LAA	Left atrial appendage
LAD	Left anterior descending artery
LCx	Left circumflex coronary artery
LIMA	Left internal mammary artery
LVAD(s)	Left ventricular assist device(s)
LVEF	Left ventricular ejection fraction
MDT	Multidisciplinary team
MPI	Myocardial perfusion imaging
MR	Mitral valve regurgitation
MRI	Magnetic resonance imaging
MV	Mitral valve
NICE	National Institute of Clinical Effectiveness
NOAC(s)	Novel oral anticoagulant(s)
OMT	Optimal medical therapy
ORACLE	Ottawa Region for Advanced Cardiovascular Research Excellence
PAF	Paroxysmal AF
PAH	Pulmonary arterial hypertension
PARTNER	Placement of aortic transcatheter valves
PCI	Percutaneous coronary intervention
PDAs	Patient decision aids
perAF	Persistent AF
PET	positron emission tomography
pLVADs	Percutaneous left ventricular devices
PV(s)	Pulmonary vein(s)
QoL	Quality of life
RCA	Right coronary artery
RCT(s)	Random controlled trial(s)/randomized clinical trial(s)
RF	Radio frequency
SA	Sinoatrial [node]
SAVR	Surgical aortic valve replacement
SCAD	Spontaneous coronary artery dissection
SCD	Sudden cardiac death
SDM	Shared decision-making
siRNA	Small interfering RNA
SPECT	Single-photon emission computed tomography
STS	Society of Thoracic Surgeons
SYNTAX	Synergy Between PCI with Taxus and Cardiac Surgery

TAA	Thoracic aortic aneurysms
TAVI	Transcatheter aortic valve implantation
TAVR	Transcatheter aortic valve replacement
TCT	Transcatheter Cardiovascular Therapeutics Symposium
TF	Transfemoral
UOHI	University of Ottawa Heart Institute
US	Ultrasound
VHD	Valvular heart disease
VT	Ventricular tachycardia
WACA	Wide antral circumferential ablation
WHH	Women's heart health

Heart Teams as a New Gold Standard of Cardiac Care

Thierry Mesana

Introduction: More Heart Teams for Better Care

In the last 10 years, with the advent of minimally invasive surgical procedures and percutaneous catheter-based approaches, the treatment of cardiac patients with valve disease has dramatically changed. Novel catheter-based devices were first presented as alternatives to conventional cardiac surgery for patients with limited life expectancy if only treated medically [1]. Most of these patients were either too old or too sick to undergo open-heart surgery. Only a few years after their initial implementation, transcatheter percutaneous valve replacement or repair is now commonly offered to the lower-risk patient population, as a valid alternative supported by large multicenter clinical trials providing clear evidence of clinical benefit. Consequently, the treatment of aortic stenosis or functional mitral regurgitation is rapidly shifting to transcatheter aortic valve implantation (TAVI) or mitral clipping (Mitraclip, Abbott Inc., USA).

Simultaneously, large randomized multicenter trials continued to feed and rejuvenate the old debate between percutaneous coronary interventions (PCIs) and coronary artery bypass graft (CABG) surgery for complex coronary artery disease (CAD).

This new paradigm in cardiac care has resulted in a different decision-making process, requiring more frequently opinions and consultations across disciplines. It has also resulted in practice changes and uncertainties for physicians, particularly those who were not early adopters.

The Heart Team concept, if well implemented, has the capacity to resolve many of these complexities and problems related to practice changes, facilitating a patient-centered approach, getting away from of a physician-centric approach which does

T. Mesana (✉)
University of Ottawa Heart Institute, Ottawa, ON, Canada
e-mail: tmesana@ottawaheart.ca

© Springer Nature Switzerland AG 2019
T. Mesana (ed.), *Heart Teams for Treatment of Cardiovascular Disease*,
https://doi.org/10.1007/978-3-030-19124-5_1

not always serve the patient best. This concept is associated with a multidisciplinary, team-based approach involving a group of cardiovascular medical experts and various healthcare professionals, each of them bringing—in a synergistic, nonsequential manner—their own level of expertise, with the ultimate goal of working together toward patient-centered care.

When the University of Ottawa Heart Institute (UOHI) conducted a survey to assess the Heart Team landscape in Canada and presented the findings at the Canadian Cardiovascular Society Annual Meeting in Montreal in October 2016, nearly half (47.6%) of the respondents to the survey indicated that their organization did not have a single heart team. However, 50% of these organizations indicated that there were plans to form a heart team.

In this survey, the majority of heart teams were reported to be organized around TAVI procedures, very few around Mitraclip. None, outside of our organization, had organized a Heart Team around CAD revascularization. Overall, the majority of Canadian centers were satisfied with their heart team(s), citing the main benefit as collaborative decision-making with shared accountability and transparency. Prior to this survey, in 2015, as part of its strategic plan, the UOHI identified the Heart Team concept as the centerpiece for delivering patient-centered cardiac care across the entire organization.

To that effect, an expanded and multiple Heart Team project was implemented gradually over a 5-year period. In addition to our Heart Transplant, TAVI, and Mitral Valve teams, we had envisioned that CAD, cardiac arrhythmias, cardiac imaging, complex critical care, and women's heart health would justify the implementation of a Heart Team concept. Our approach was not only to focus on procedures or diseases, but also to build new teams around wider themes addressing issues unresolved by our current models of care in cardiac imaging or critical care. Even more specific was our initiative of a Women's Heart Health (WHH) team, which was addressing a broader healthcare issue rather than a disease-specific focus.

As quoted from the Chap. 7, "The issues affecting the field of women's cardiovascular health are distinctly different from those being addressed by current Heart Teams, as providers working in this field are faced with a relative paucity of scientific data to drive clinical decisions, in addition to low levels of awareness and education about the unique aspects of cardiovascular disease in women." Our WHH Heart Team has been rapidly impactful within our organization and community, generating new ideas, disseminating new research, and attracting large external financial support. This team has contributed to reinforce gender equity and female leadership within our organization, creating a significant momentum, so that Women's Heart Health has become a top strategic priority for the next 5 years.

For our cardiac arrhythmias team, the focus was decided to be on atrial fibrillation (AF). A comprehensive heart team focused on patient selection, procedural improvements, and continuum of care was designed to be superior to a standard electrophysiology team, restricted to cardiologists specialized in catheter-based AF ablations. Indeed, the addition of heart failure cardiologists, cardiac surgeons, and hematologists added a new dimension to the care of AF patients, harmonized

anticoagulation protocols, and opened the door to novel ideas such as regional AF triage model or hybrid AF procedures, to be done jointly by electrophysiologists and dedicated cardiac surgeons.

This book includes a variety of chapters that can help healthcare organizations starting or expanding heart teams in different areas, including in less common themes, as above cited. We did not pretend to explore all domains of cardiac care which could potentially benefit from the Heart Team concept. Each center should actually decide to build its own multiple Heart Team program based on its own needs to improve care, enhance patient satisfaction, and maximize hospital efficiency. We do not provide a magic solution to the risk of failure of any particular team. In any case, multiple heart teams should be built strategically and gradually, engaging the right people properly and managing timing as well as the risk of failure.

Building Multiple Heart Teams Is Challenging

Healthcare teams are more complicated than non-healthcare teams, and team models from other professions or domains may not be easily transferable to healthcare [2]. While implementing our multiple Heart Team project, we encountered various levels of difficulties. Clearly, some teams were faster in achieving their full potential than others, while other ones found it challenging to establish common goals and objectives. Regularly cited as impeding the performance of heart teams are the logistical difficulties coordinating schedules and physician availability. Other significant challenges are related to financial aspects such as physician billing, level of funding for procedures, and administrative support, or related to infrastructure such as adequate meeting rooms or access to hybrid operating rooms.

Last but not least, cardiac programs may not have access to an adequate data warehouse with dedicated databases, including follow-up to monitor results beyond 1 month postprocedure. Too often, the only way to get long-term data is through large regional or national administrative data warehouses. Those are important and helpful in many ways, but not easy to access, and lack granularity, missing discrete data to evaluate complex cardiac procedures. To better help heart teams, a coordinated effort is necessary, developing comprehensive research databases linked to advanced health information systems. Participation in international registries should also be contemplated for teams involved in novel devices implantation, such as TAVI.

Quite challenging, in our experience as for many others, was the "cultural" barrier and resistance to move away from a "specialty-oriented" historical culture between cardiologists and surgeons. Competition between services was a predictable issue, even in a center like the UOHI, with a 40-year history of a collegial, team-based Heart Institute model. Although the Heart Team concept was reinforced in Guidelines of Revascularization of CAD, following Syntax Trials [3, 4], it was still challenging to convince the same UOHI cardiologists taking part of well-functioning TAVI or Mitraclip teams to adhere to a CAD Heart Team imposing a significant cultural change.

Indeed, our CAD Heart Team required more time to design the right process for patients falling into the "gray zone," such as those presenting with triple vessel disease, left main disease, or diabetic patients. Organizing a team review right after an angiogram or even within 24 hours was logistically difficult. Coordinating schedules was challenging, even if most cardiac surgeons and interventional cardiologists agreed on and valued the team model. The Heart Team concept for CAD patients was perceived by some as an impractical concept and inefficient management of resources. Indeed, taking a patient off the table and waiting for a team review can be inefficient and an inconvenience if the patient ends up having a PCI and not a CABG.

Even stable patients would most likely favor ad-hoc PCI if they are asked while still on the table. However, this would prevent them from giving a well-informed consent and to eventually benefit from a team instead of individual approach.

In light of our experience, we believe that the first step for the CAD Heart team should be to agree on the principle of an institutional approach limiting variations of practice in coronary revascularization, avoiding "self-referral." Ideally, the CAD Heart Team should discuss and agree first on indications and options for stable CAD by both interventional cardiologists and cardiac surgeons. Harmonizing the views and opinions can be achieved through a constructive dialog guided by science, data, and mutual respect. The team would then establish a simple process to review within less than 24 hours for patients in the "gray zone," based on the Syntax score and clinical information from the referring physicians. Finally, patients would be provided with clear explanations, so they would better understand the details of each procedure and the aspects related to immediate and long-term results, and choose one technique vs. another in an unbiased fashion. This would apply both ways, as cardiac surgeons may refer patients directly, who could actually benefit from PCI instead of CABG. Finally, although differences exist between countries or even hospitals within the same country or region [5], it should not prevent CAD teams to be effective, regardless of logistical or other factors unrelated to patients.

Helpful to the necessary cultural change can be the promotion of new team projects such as hybrid revascularization that are performed in a hybrid OR, involving members who complete each other and not compete against each other. An essential goal of the team should also be to collect PCI and CABG in the same database with common definitions and detailed follow-up.

Cultural barriers may also be observed while implementing a Cardiac Imaging Heart Team. It can be challenging to closely bring two specialties such as cardiology and radiology, potentially competing for same resources. Different modalities require different training, background, and expertise such as CT, MRI, echocardiography, PET, PET/MR, or nuclear imaging. Those technologies evolve quickly and constantly, becoming more or less obsolete or redundant. These changes put significant pressure on the hospital budget and capital equipment planning.

Patient waitlists can also be mismanaged due to a lack of clinical coordination or communication between units or departments. Hence, the best way to get the "right test at the right time for the right patient" is to build a Cardiac Imaging Heart Team, including cardiologists, radiologists, and biomedical and IT engineers. In addition,

data scientists are highly desirable to develop artificial intelligence through the development of algorithms and machine learning. The team should address important questions related to which modalities should be combined in hybrid imaging, avoiding redundant tests. There should be a clear benefit of a team approach for the development of multimodality imaging and hybrid imaging platforms more particularly.

Similarly, building a Critical Care Team involving intensivists, cardiologists, and surgeons is challenging, although it should necessarily lead to a better approach for acutely ill patients. Cardiac centers such as UOHI require large intensive-care resources, the majority of these resources being dedicated to a minority of patients. At UOHI, about 20% of our surgical patients, the sickest ones, occupy about 80% of our total bed capacity. Furthermore, we are seeing a clear trend of patients in the cardiology intensive care unit (ICU) looking like our surgical patients. Like in the cardiac surgical ICU, more cardiology ICU patients require advanced life support, such as renal replacement therapy, artificial ventilation, or mechanical circulatory support. Complex patients, such as those with advanced heart failure, acute cardiogenic shock, or out-of-hospital cardiac arrest, are referred to cardiology ICUs. We often see critically ill patients in the cardiology ICU after high-risk catheter-based procedures, or waiting for heart transplant on heavy life-support management. Comprehensive Critical Cardiac Care teams are definitely a critical, strategic initiative, leading to harmonized management for critical care across the entire organization. Such patients need to be managed by highly specialized healthcare professionals assembled in a dedicated team. This implies creating a group of Cardiac Intensivists working closely with cardiologists and cardiac surgeons at various steps, including patient selection and preparation for procedures, or implementation of emergency protocols and codes for various situations. The team should implement and evaluate new therapies in a similar way for all ICUs.

Finally, dedicated ICU databases with similar data definition and follow-up should be developed for administrative and research purposes, monitoring efficiencies, complications, and outcomes, and sharing data in regular multidisciplinary meetings including staff and trainees.

Heart Teams for Better Care at Less Cost

Financial considerations often impede the development of heart teams. They fall into two broad categories: organizational support and financial reimbursement models. Both are interrelated. In order for heart teams to influence care delivery, dedicated financial support is needed from funding agencies to hospitals. Funding for procedures comes with accountability for outcomes. For instance, heart teams are a requirement for TAVI reimbursement by Medicare in the United States. In Ontario, the definition of heart teams for TAVI is becoming increasingly important to determine specific volume allocation for each center. Therefore, it is likely that the demonstration of a true, effective Heart Team model become a prerequisite to support funding of novel, high-cost cardiac procedures. Regardless of the healthcare

funding system, entirely public, private, or mixed, governments and health insurance companies are increasingly interested in linking funding to outcomes and quality measurement to reimbursement. Consequently, funding models will trend inevitably toward bundled payments and value-added delivery model. Heart teams will be essential to adjust funding to complex patient care pathways. For instance, instead of funding a program separately for the number of TAVI procedures vs. the number of surgical aortic valve replacements, cardiac centers should be funded for treating an adequate number of patients presenting aortic valve stenosis and requiring intervention. It would be up to the heart team to decide what is best for each patient and to implement the best care possible. Heart teams would be responsible for reducing procedure times, in-hospital complications, and follow-up after discharge up to 3 months or even a year in certain cases. Bundled payment should include rehabilitation and remote monitoring, as they will likely benefit patients, reduce readmissions, and improve medication compliance and quality of life. These measures should lead to better quality care, cost reduction, and higher patient satisfaction.

Similarly, for CAD, a heart team could have a major role in a bundled payment system if funding could be delivered based on quality and outcomes including 1-year follow-up for both PCI and CABG. For cardiac imaging, the impact of a team organizing a cohesive centralized, patient-centered intake could eliminate up to 30% of costs due to test redundancy. These savings would be huge, helping hospitals to invest in new technology or equipment updates, or research in cardiac imaging. One could imagine a bundled cardiac imaging payment for diagnostic, with adjusters depending upon a variety of conditions or procedures requiring additional testing.

Finally, in many countries such as Canada or United States, physicians are paid on fees for service, designed for delivering procedures with little accountability for appropriateness. A new model could include a bundle payment for physician's fees together with the bundled hospital payment as an incentive to engage all stakeholders to improve quality and efficiency with less costs and more access to care. By not being paid or funded *in silos*, hospitals and Heart Teams could work together to provide better care at less cost.

Heart Teams are Superior for Education and Knowledge Translation

Heart Teams also have the ability to significantly transform education and high-level training, not only across medical specialties, but also across multiple healthcare professions. The combination of new cardiovascular technology with increasing patient complexity brings physicians and trainees from different specialties together, breaking down traditional silos. There is a great deal of knowledge to acquire together as a team and disseminate to others.

Nowadays, surgeons are eager to perform less-invasive procedures, are becoming more familiar with advanced intraoperative imaging, and are acquiring catheter

skills. At the same time, interventional cardiologists are acquiring more knowledge of valve disease management in terms of echocardiographic imaging or complex postoperative care and benefit from decades of surgical experience of the anatomical and physiological challenges observed in various valve replacement or repair procedures. Actually, a number of innovative percutaneous solutions reproduce techniques widely used in the surgical field, such as mitral valve clipping or annular remodeling. Similarly, a TAVI reproduces a surgical aortic valve replacement, with a much less-invasive approach but with similar complications, such as complete heart block requiring a pacemaker implant, prosthetic leakages or deterioration leading to valve dysfunction. The same issues of residual mitral valve regurgitation and long-term stability of functional result are observed both in surgical and in catheter-based implantations.

For AF, cardiac surgeons performing AF ablation procedures observe more or less the same patterns of AF recurrence as cardiologists experience in catheter-based AF ablation.

More practice and knowledge sharing across cardiac specialties inevitably adds value. Heart teams should have the mandate to educate with cross-training, engaging staff and trainees in evidence-based guidelines and clinical research.

Furthermore, heart teams are best positioned to develop implementation of hub-and-spoke models. With the advancement of remote monitoring and virtual clinic, heart teams will play a key role to the coordination of care outside hospital walls. For instance, heart failure teams can use telemedicine to enhance the training of colleagues in partner hospitals, so patients in remote areas would receive expert level care close to home.

Finally, medical schools need to better adapt their curriculum to innovation in care delivery. Heart teams offer more opportunities for new leaders and teachers to be promoting a different model of medical education. In the chapter on Cardiac Imaging, the authors advance the concept of a "Cardiac Imaging Virtual University" to promote an Internet-based high-quality education.

Is There a Standard Heart Team Model?

We do not believe that there is a singular model for heart team development. Successful heart teams always manage to build a culture of trust and dialog, putting patients first. In order to address specific challenges, each team must adapt and eventually change management. To reduce the risk of failure, right decisions are needed around leadership and membership, both critical to optimize team performance. Constant team development is also important to consider. Undeniably, Heart Institutes or similar dedicated heart centers have an advantage and should lead the way. They are large facilities, usually partnering with large academic hospitals, with a mission based on three pillars: patient care, research, and education. They have the necessary critical mass of cross-disciplinary cardiac experts, working together for years, sharing a history of common accomplishments. They treat large numbers of complex patients through a wide regional referral base, sometimes extending

nationally or internationally. Dedicated heart centers have a governance and leadership structure with the ability to strategically allocate funds to their teams. Cardiac programs depending on large, multilayered hospital administrations have lesser financial autonomy and control. Large hospitals may be facing multiple priorities and various budget constraints in areas other than cardiac care. It then becomes harder for cardiac specialists to implement and pioneer cardiac innovations or build new models of cardiac care.

Academic hospitals are also structured around multiple divisions under respective departments which may not spontaneously favor cross-fertilization between specialties. The Heart Team concept is facilitated by a governance model allowing physicians to think beyond their specialty, more synergistically, and with the administration actually providing the resources dedicated to patient-centered care. Although there is not one single model of heart teams, they need to follow terms of reference including a common set of deliverables and be truly interprofessional (physicians, nurses, allied health). They need to be given a broad mandate and adaptability, which includes developing novel strategies, such as hub-and-spoke activities, offering educational and leadership opportunities, and promoting collaborative clinical research across specialties. Heart teams should have clear leadership built in, either medical and surgical co-leadership or following a dyad model including a physician and a high-level administrator. The group should meet at its own pace, with its own agenda, depending on goals chosen collectively. A project coordinator is fundamental at all phases, facilitating team building, monitoring recurrent issues, and helping with change management as needed.

At UOHI, each heart team reports directly to the administration's senior management. Implementing heart teams should be a "learn as we go" experience requiring significant institutional support. As part of the UOHI overall administrative support, we have been building an innovative institutional database platform, named "Cardiocore" consisting of a complex but comprehensive modular dataset, to allow heart teams to be collecting information across the full spectrum of care for all patients undergoing cardiac procedures, including long-term follow-up.

Conclusion

It was a major practice shift when, at the very start of the TAVI experience, interventional cardiologists and cardiac surgeons started working side by side during procedures, assisting each other like colleagues belonging to the same specialty. This was a true game changer in cardiac care, not only for cardiologists and surgeons, but also for many others and for patients first. In a previous article [6] we wrote that Heart Teams were a new paradigm and a new era for cardiac care. The Heart Team concept has called cardiac centers to a profound rethinking of the current models of care, forcing healthcare leaders to be thinking out of the box and looking at a bigger

picture. Heart teams which were built to deliver catheter-based valve therapy are now paving the way to expand the Heart Team concept to deliver patient-centered care everywhere. In addition, heart teams will allow for the emergence of a new generation of cardiac experts, a hybrid type of specialist between cardiac surgeons and interventional cardiologists, with a new set of skills.

This "new world" needs to be well understood and promoted by healthcare administrators, funding organizations, policy makers, and academic leaders, encouraging and supporting these teams across hospitals, heart institutes, and departments.

The research impact will be significant, as Heart Teams form a critical mass of investigators generating new ideas and creating new forums for multidisciplinary groups. As described in this book, UOHI linked heart teams to innovation hubs in various themes such as valve disease, heart failure, or cardiac arrhythmias and used women's heart health as a crosscutting theme across these themes. Moreover, heart teams such as cardiac imaging or critical care have the capacity to integrate data solutions and data linkages, and develop a holistic model of artificial intelligence serving the patients first. Although these potential benefits of heart teams still need to be quantified and validated at a larger scale, we trust that early adopters will create a new gold standard model for care for decades to come.

References

1. Leon MB, Smith CR, Mack M, Miller DC, Moses JW, Svensson LG, et al. Transcatheter aortic-valve implantation for aortic stenosis in patients who cannot undergo surgery. N Engl J Med. 2010;363(17):1597–607.
2. Andreatta PB. A typology of healthcare teams. Health Care Manage Rev. 2010;35(4):345–54.
3. Patel MR, Calhoon JH, Dehmer GJ, Grantham JA, Maddox TM, Maron DJ, et al. ACC/AATS/AHA/ASE/ASNC/SCAI/SCCT/STS 2017 appropriate use criteria for coronary revascularization in patients with stable ischemic heart disease: a report of the American College of Cardiology Appropriate use Criteria Task Force, American Association for Thoracic Surgery, American Heart Association, American Society of Echocardiography, American Society of Nuclear Cardiology, Society for Cardiovascular Angiography and Interventions, Society of Cardiovascular Computed Tomography, and Society of Thoracic Surgeons. J Am Coll Cardiol. 2017;69(17):2212–41.
4. Windecker S, Kolh P, Alfonso F, Collet JP, Cremer J, Falk V, Filippatos G, et al. 2014 ESC/EACTS guidelines on myocardial revascularization: the task force on myocardial revascularization of the European Society of Cardiology (ESC) and the European Association for Cardio-Thoracic Surgery (EACTS) developed with the special contribution of the European Association of Percutaneous Cardiovascular Interventions (EAPCI). Eur Heart J. 2014;35(37):2541–619.
5. Lemay M, Wells GA, Choung AY. Do the results of the SYNTAX trial apply to my center? EuroIntervention. 2017;13(7):781–3.
6. Mesana T, Rodger N, Sherrard H. Heart teams: a new paradigm in healthcare. Can J Cardiol. 2018;34(7):815–8.

Complex Coronary Revascularization Heart Team

2

Aun-Yeong Chong, Terry Meadows, and David Glineur

Illustrative Case

A 66-year-old male with previous percutaneous coronary intervention (PCI) to the mid left anterior descending (LAD) artery and mid right coronary artery (RCA) in 1999 was referred to a diagnostic cardiologist for coronary angiogram following a myocardial perfusion scan as part of preoperative workup for management of an incidental distal esophageal T2N0 adenocarcinoma. A *curative* esophagectomy was intended as there was no evidence of regional nodal or distant metastatic disease. The myocardial perfusion scan demonstrated a large area of ischemia in the entire inferolateral territory, moderate-sized area of ischemia in the mid anterior, and apex accounting for 27% of the left ventricular mass. Left ventricular ejection fraction was normal. His cardiovascular risk factors included previous smoking, hypertension, dyslipidemia, and type 2 diabetes mellitus.

Coronary angiography demonstrated restenosis of both the previously stented LAD and RCA. In addition, there was a severe stenosis in the proximal LAD in continuity with the previously stented mid LAD that also had a long segment of stenosis. The patient was referred to the Complex Revascularization Heart Team for review and decision on the optimal strategy. The SYNTAX score was calculated to be 30, with a Euroscore II of 1.5%. In the presence of diabetes, a superior medium- to long-term outcome would be expected with coronary artery bypass graft surgery (CABG) compared to PCI. In the absence of the adenocarcinoma, CABG would

A.-Y. Chong (✉)
University of Ottawa Heart Institute, Department of Cardiology, Ottawa, ON, Canada
e-mail: achong@ottawaheart.ca

T. Meadows
University of Ottawa Heart Institute, Ottawa, ON, Canada

D. Glineur
Cardiac Surgery, University of Ottawa Heart Institute, Ottawa, ON, Canada

© Springer Nature Switzerland AG 2019
T. Mesana (ed.), *Heart Teams for Treatment of Cardiovascular Disease*,
https://doi.org/10.1007/978-3-030-19124-5_2

have been the guideline recommended revascularization strategy. It was also the opinion of the anesthetist that the cardiac risk was significant, and revascularization should be undertaken first with neoadjuvant chemotherapy administered in the recovery period to contain the adenocarcinoma. A combined CABG and esophagectomy was also proposed but ultimately rejected as the treatment of choice.

As the timing was crucial to minimize the risk of metastasis, a strategy to expedite recovery was needed. With the local expertise available, a hybrid revascularization strategy with minimally invasive left internal mammary artery (LIMA) to LAD and diagonal artery through a left anterior thoracotomy and subsequent PCI of the RCA were performed, attaining complete revascularization expeditiously. This allowed the patient to undergo neoadjuvant chemotherapy, laparoscopic staging that excluded any evidence of peritoneal carcinomatosis, and eventually thoracoscopic esophagectomy with clear resection margins in the next 3 months. However, the patient died from unexpected omental and peritoneal metastatic esophageal adenocarcinoma 8 months later.

Despite the unfortunate outcome of the patient, this case illustrates the importance of a multidisciplinary team approach. One could argue that PCI would have been the preferred strategy, but that would have necessitated dual antiplatelet therapy and the risk of stent thrombosis perioperatively with temporary interruption of at least one antiplatelet agent. The mortality risk to the patient should this occur in the proximal LAD would have been substantial. Had the outcome of the esophageal adenocarcinoma been favorable, the long-term benefit of LIMA to LAD would have been realized, granted it remains to be seen if that still held true with a hybrid approach. The SYNTAX score would have also predicted a superior outcome with the complexity of coronary artery disease (CAD), notwithstanding the diabetic status.

Introduction

The concept of a multidisciplinary team's role in an individual patient is not new, but more entrenched in some medical specialties such as oncology, elderly care, and radiology, more so than others. It is essential in improving the quality of care. Its introduction into routine practice in other medical specialties such as adult cardiology has been met with greater resistance. In the era of randomized controlled trials of coronary revascularization and percutaneous valve procedures, discussions by "heart teams" are a prerequisite for randomization to ascertain equipoise between the treatment arms. However, this has not translated into widespread acceptance in daily clinical practice. This could be due to the often-perceived antagonistic relationship between cardiac surgeons and interventional cardiologists, or the paternalistic culture within cardiology itself that "the doctor knows best." In the current era where trial evidence is emerging at exponential speed, and careful evaluation and application to specific patient groups is required, the concept of a single physician making decisions in complex cases becomes ever more difficult, and sometimes indefensible, in the event of medical errors. It also denies the patient of choice when two different approaches to treatment are indeed equivalent.

The 2017 Appropriate Use Criteria for Coronary Revascularization in Patients with Stable Ischemic Heart Disease [1] strongly recommends a heart team approach in patients with unprotected left main and complex CAD. In addition, the 2018 ESC/EACTS Guidelines on myocardial revascularization states that active patient participation in the decision-making process should be encouraged and that evidence-based information should be provided and uncertainties associated with different treatment strategies discussed using terminology that is easily understood by patients [2]. The need for a heart team is underlined by reports of either under-use, or inappropriate use, of optimal revascularization strategies, with wide variation between countries and even hospitals within the same vicinity. A recent report from Canada in 2014 demonstrated that even within the province of Ontario, there was a wide variation in revascularization strategies for patients with multivessel disease that cannot be explained by different coronary anatomical complexity as measured by SYNTAX score, with PCI:CABG ratio ranging from 0.24 to 5.00 [3]. Similar disparities have also been published in Europe [2]. This could be due to several reasons, including variations in interpretation of complexity and severity of coronary anatomy that is influenced by the culture at individual institutions [3]. It could also reflect a difference in the availability of local expertise and results from different revascularization strategies.

A multidisciplinary approach can minimize specialty bias between cardiac surgery and interventional cardiology and prevent self-referral from interfering with optimal patient care. Perhaps, this is more applicable to interventional cardiology than cardiac surgery, as diagnostic coronary angiograms are often performed by the same operator and thus seen as the "gatekeepers" to cardiac surgery. In fee-for-service healthcare models, this can be misconstrued as a financial conflict of interest, even if small financial "penalties" are imposed for combined diagnostic and interventional procedures performed at the same sitting.

Mandate of the Coronary Revascularization Heart Team

The Coronary Revascularization Heart Team is tasked with the evaluation of patients where revascularization is indicated and appropriate for complex CAD, where an immediate decision is not required. Criteria based on current evidence have been formulated to identify patients with complex CAD in particular, but not exclusive to, multivessel CAD with or without left ventricular dysfunction, patients with CAD and diabetes mellitus and left main coronary artery stenosis. This is to avoid unnecessary referrals where data supports PCI as the preferred treatment in very large-volume centers.

In stable ischemic heart disease (IHD), it should be recognized that PCI is not associated with improved survival when compared with optimal medical therapy (OMT). While ad hoc PCI is still performed in most cases and has been demonstrated to be safe [4], it provides less opportunity for patients and their physicians to thoughtfully consider a range of clinically equivalent treatment options after the coronary anatomy is known. It is interesting to note that when patients with stronger indications for CABG underwent coronary angiography in hospitals without the

ability to perform ad hoc PCI, patients were more likely to be recommended CABG [5]. This immediately raises the probable bias, as it is unlikely that the patient and physician would choose a more invasive treatment, i.e., CABG, if PCI would have conferred the same outcome.

The demonstration of complex CAD by coronary angiography should prompt a pause to allow further evaluation not just of the coronary anatomy but of the patient as a whole, such as concomitant illness, frailty, quality of life, life expectancy, and patient preference. There is robust data to support the use of the SYNTAX score [6] to guide revascularization strategy, with CABG conferring a mortality benefit with more complex disease as defined by intermediate to high SYNTAX scores, such that it is accorded a class IIa recommendation by the relevant bodies to aid decision-making [1]. However, the calculation of the SYNTAX score is not instantaneous and requires trained personnel who perform it routinely and systematically so that the rules for scoring lesions are adhered strictly for it to be valid. It should also be recognized that there is inter- and intra-observer variability in calculating the SYNTAX score, but this can be minimized with continual training and validation [7–11]. In addition, the STS and EuroSCORE II are calculated in order to assess the surgical risk of the patient. Often, critical pieces of information are unavailable to the treating interventional cardiologist, especially when patients are referred from external hospitals and the interventional cardiologist is only meeting the patient for the first time. While shared electronic medical records may be a solution to some of these problems, often, hospital medical records are incomplete, and a history obtained in a hurry from the patient is unreliable.

While it is tempting for the treating interventional cardiologist to perform ad hoc PCI to avoid a separate procedure and arterial access with its inherent risk, it deprives the patient of the opportunity to discuss options of treatment with full disclosure of available information following coronary angiography. It is true that some patients would prefer the "doctor knows best" approach of a single physician-centric decision-maker; it is often ethically and medicolegally challenging when the patient has been given sedation and insufficient time to consider, the analogy being able to walk away to gather more information before making a choice when making a purchase of large household appliances. In this situation, patients are denied the opportunity to question the risk/benefit ratio of the treatment and even the offer of a second opinion. In addition, there is no "cooling-off" period in ad hoc PCI, as the treatment cannot be reversed. By referring and discussing such patients within the context of the heart team, other opinions are considered, and consensus can be attained as to the best approach. In addition, when the discussion revolves around CABG versus PCI, one could legitimately argue that the surgeon is not qualified on his own to provide the patient with the most up-to-date information and how the PCI procedure would be performed. The converse is also true of the interventional cardiologist providing a surgical opinion. This is pertinent in the current era when patients may have access to the individualized physician complication rates.

Members of the Coronary Revascularization Heart Team

The Coronary Revascularization Heart Team should comprise a minimum of one interventional cardiologist, one cardiac surgeon, and a noninterventional cardiologist to be quorate [12]. The presence of a noninterventional cardiologist should be encouraged, as this will reduce the risk of bias. It is also beneficial to have the referring physician who knows the patient well present key points related to the patient that may impact on the decision-making process. Other members may include clerical personnel to document the main points of discussion, the final decision regarding revascularization as appropriate, and by which strategy (PCI versus CABG). It is also important that the patient is preferably referred to the interventional cardiologist or cardiac surgeon who is present in order to avoid second- or even third-hand information and, consequently, a difference in opinion. Those present would have discussed not just the coronary anatomy but the comorbidities of the patient and any other nuances that are not appreciated by a physician who does not know the patient well. Hence, it is vital that the cardiologist most responsible for the patient is present as the patient's advocate so that the best possible decision is made. Unfortunately, this is often impossible due to physicians' schedules.

On a broader scale as in the case of our Coronary Revascularization Heart Team, the team also includes nurse educators, nurse practitioners, triage personnel, cardiac anesthetist, and a clinical psychologist. The role of this expanded team of experts includes the education of patients and their family members before and after the revascularization procedures. Addressing issues early on such as the need for postdischarge care expedites the discharge process, and a social package can be planned either in advance or at the time of patient admission.

Benefits of the Revascularization Heart Team

To the Patient

The patient benefits from a more considered approach to the management of his or her disease, allowing time for adequate discussion. It is important to emphasize that immediate revascularization, in most cases percutaneously, is not mandatory. The recently published ORBITA trial if anything has proven that despite what is accepted as physiologically significant disease, a delay of several weeks while uptitrating medications did not cause harm [13]. In patients with moderately complex CAD as defined by intermediate SYNTAX scores, an informed discussion should be compulsory, as although a mortality benefit was shown in the SYNTAX trial when patients underwent CABG, the benefit was more modest. Some patients may have reasons to prefer PCI, for example, expedited return to work or other concomitant illness that require expedited recovery. On the other hand, patients may have true allergy or severe adverse reactions to antiplatelet agents, thereby favoring CABG. Such information is often not immediately available, as the patient may have only been started on the medications on the day of or shortly before the

procedure itself. Moreover, it is not unusual that the physician performing coronary angiography is not the patient's usual physician.

In addition, the patient should also have greater confidence that the correct management has been recommended and his or her case has been discussed by a team of specialists and not just a solitary physician with inherent bias [14].

To the Team Members

By having frequent discussions across the subspecialties, team members learn the subtleties of proposed revascularization procedures. The exchange of experience and trial data between the cardiac surgeon, interventional cardiologist, imaging cardiologist, and cardiac anesthetist must be advantageous. The presence of a non-interventional cardiologist is preferred so that bias toward one strategy over another where evidence is equivocal is tempered. Where there is an absence of robust evidence available to determine the management of a patient, consensus and shared responsibility should be achieved. This also becomes fertile ground for the generation of research ideas.

To the Health System

By determining the management strategy based on relevant trial data and discussion between the Revascularization Heart Team and the patient's physician, it is more likely that the best possible decision is made for the individual patient. By considering the patient's comorbidities and frailty, one could potentially avoid a more invasive procedure which may not prolong the patient's life but result in prolonged hospital stay, necessitating higher costs to the health system. Selection of inappropriate patients for CABG may lead to extended stays in the intensive care unit and the requirement of extracorporeal circulatory support, which can be prohibitively expensive and contraindicated.

Challenges Experienced by the Coronary Revascularization Heart Team

The biggest challenge has been the change of practice away from ad hoc PCI. Most interventional cardiologists still deem this to be the best management strategy to avoid a second procedure and second arterial access, which carry its own complications. In addition, the logistics of rebooking the patient onto another list on a later date often causes inconvenience to the patient and triage office. This may lead to patient dissatisfaction, but it is mainly the management of the patient's expectation. If patients are informed early on that their coronary angiogram may not lead to immediate treatment should further discussion be required when more complex disease than expected is encountered, most are appreciative that extra consideration is being taken in their interest.

There is also a move away from a single physician-centric decision-maker or even a single physician to a single surgeon model, to a team-based approach in intermediate to complex CAD. In a perfect setting, the Coronary Revascularization

Heart Team meeting should have several interventional cardiologists and several cardiac surgeons to discuss the best strategy, especially in very complex patients. Differing opinions should be voiced and supported by evidence rather than anecdotal personal experience. In addition, even among interventional cardiologists and cardiac surgeons, certain skill sets exist within individuals that are not common to the group. Among interventional cardiologists, it may be PCI of chronic total occlusions, advanced interpretation of intravascular imaging, or use of coronary physiology or familiarity with other ancillary equipment such as laser or rotational atherectomy as well as mechanical circulatory support. Among cardiac surgeons, it may be the options of off-pump surgery, minimally invasive bypass surgery, total arterial bypass grafting, or robotic-assisted surgery. Finally, a hybrid revascularization approach could also be considered in appropriate settings. It certainly requires setting aside egos and recognizing one's limitations, as being able to perform a procedure does not equate to another individual who has performed the procedure numerous times with lower complication rates. This is particularly relevant in countries where individual physician outcomes are in public domain (e.g. United Kingdom [12]) and informed patients may request a particular physician. Even though it is not the intention of releasing such data to the public, the data needs to be interpreted with guidance, as it does not encompass every procedure or operation, especially if exceptionally high risk. Patients may need explanation that a very skilled physician taking on the higher-risk operation may have a worse outcome. This is the basis of the argument to publish institutional, rather than individual, data.

Other challenges essential to the implementation of an effective heart team are facilities and administrative support. A room with the facility to display all cardiac-imaging modalities (CT, MRI, nuclear imaging, echocardiograms, and coronary angiograms) and access to other relevant investigations are required to enable the process to run smoothly. The ability to hold teleconferences in the room so that physicians can participate remotely is crucial, especially to enable contact with the physician who knows the patient best. The technology is available, but would require the local Information Technology departmental support and associated costs.

At the end of the process, the patient and his or her physician will need to be informed of the outcome and schedule either for the procedure or a clinic visit to discuss further, whereupon a truly informed consent can be obtained. This will require the support of clerical staff to maintain the crucial link. Documentation of the discussion needs to include the salient points leading to the decision so that it can be revisited in future. Clerical staff is also essential to gather the relevant results of investigations and risk scores to inform the heart team.

Barriers Hindering the Coronary Revascularization Heart Team from Performing at Full Potential

The main barrier to a multidisciplinary team approach for revascularization is the entrenched mindset of cardiac surgeons being mere technicians and seen as

competition rather than complementary to the management of complex patients. Traditionally, the management of the complex patient has been in the hands of cardiologists who know the patient well, leading to the label of "gatekeepers," appropriately or not. This can be contentious in the current era of "revolving door" hospitalizations and day-case procedures whereby very little time is spent speaking to the patient and the patient's family about the disease and its management. Very limited time is available for discussion, and hence, multiple booklets and pamphlets are produced to "inform" the patient, but such an approach paints every patient with the same broad brush. Often patients or their family will search the Internet for information that is inappropriate or simply wrong, as there are very few safeguards to the veracity of data available online. Scientific journals are often limited to the public due to prohibitive subscription fees, and are also beyond rational interpretation by the lay public. This sometimes creates unnecessary tension and mistrust toward the physician.

While the interventional cardiologist has a duty of care to the patient to determine what is best for the patient, the cardiac surgeon has an identical role to be equally involved in engaging discussions and management of the patient. Combined rounds, be it clinical or continuing medical education, are a rarity, and both groups tend to work in silos. Constant debate when new evidence arises that challenges current practice is not only healthy to promote discussion, but also highlights where evidence-free zones are for future research, especially within academic centers, which are supposed to be the beacons of best practice. Colleagues may deem their clinical acumen beyond reproach, and such attitudes need to be tempered by the fact that when a malpractice lawsuit prevails, the reputation of the institute is at stake, not merely the individual's. In such a situation, the fact that the decision was made by a committee of experts may mitigate the risk to an extent.

In addition to the needed change in local mindset, it is unfortunate that "fee-for-service" healthcare models reimburse procedures far more lucratively than the cognitive efforts involved in discussion of complex patients, leading to the belief that it is not worth the physicians' time. As such, the attendance at heart team meetings should ideally be incorporated into the consultant physicians' job plans [12] as it is an essential part of clinical care, even if it is not remunerated. Scheduling of heart team meetings, especially in larger centers, needs to be commensurate with the volume so that each meeting is not overwhelmed with too many patients so that the participants become fatigued at the end. In larger centers, it may need to be at least twice a week, if not more.

How Is the Heart Team Measuring Success?

"The proof of the pudding is in the eating." If the process is not adopted widely by affiliated groups, then it becomes futile. Both patient and physician need to recognize that the process is worth its while so that the right decision is made. Ultimately, the measure of success needs to be the improved outcome for patients. In this respect, there is currently a lack of published data. Complex patients represent only

a minority of cases within each establishment, and a concerted effort is required for data collection over a number of years in order to prove that not only the process led to the correct management of the patient based on risk assessment predictors but that the decision led to a more favorable long-term outcome which in terms of CABG over PCI requires at the very minimum 5 years of follow-up. Consistency and reproducibility of heart team decisions have been demonstrated by other centers [15, 16], but need to be replicated locally.

Lessons Learned in Establishing a Revascularization Heart Team

While it may seem obvious from the beginning, the establishment of a heart team requires individuals with a common mindset and the tenacity to implement changes that appear to impede optimal patient care. Furthermore, the rewards are not to these individuals necessarily, but hopefully to patients. In fact, being a proponent of a shared decision-making model is often interpreted as a sign of weakness. While "Rome was not built in a day," the successful establishment of the heart team may be more tedious, as the implementation requires cajoling and convincing of physicians that it is the better way, and that a team is always better than an individual when making difficult decisions. This must be done diplomatically and not antagonistically.

The necessary support by hospital administrators is key to the process, as physician time needs to be recognized and, if possible, compensated. There is also a need for legal representation highlighting the exposure of the physician and institution to the risk of malpractice in this era of an increasingly litigious society and how a multidisciplinary approach may mitigate that. Often it is not that the right decision has been made, but the need to be seen doing so that matters.

The ultimate beneficiary of this process is the patient; engaging patient advocate groups may be needed to convince their physicians. This may be more effective in a system where the patient has a choice of physicians.

What Does the Future Look Like?

The time of the multidisciplinary team approach in managing complex patients is already here, like it or not. With the abundant trials being published, it is impossible for individual physicians to synthesize all the information. Within the revascularization heart team, data that may influence decision-making comes from cardiac imaging, interventional cardiology, cardiac surgery, and even anesthesiology. With greater emphasis on coronary physiology by invasive and noninvasive means, the interpretation of such data is paramount in guiding decision-making. The recognition of addressing factors that influence the success of patient management (e.g., glycemic control, lipid management, antiplatelet management, perioperative management) and the importance of assessing frailty is such that no single physician can do it all, nor has the expertise to do so.

More recently, the SYNTAX score II that incorporates clinical variables into the anatomical SYNTAX score to predict 4-year mortality for both CABG and PCI has begun to show promise, and would predictably be used to guide future decision-making by the heart team [17–20]. Longer term is needed. SYNTAX III Revolution is an interesting trial randomizing two heart teams to select between CABG and PCI according to either invasive coronary angiography or noninvasive cardiac CT, guided by the SYNTAX score II and FFR derived from coronary CT angiography [20, 21]. If shown to be positive, the role of the invasive diagnostic cardiologist and by extension, the interventional cardiologist, performing diagnostic coronary angiography as the gatekeeper to revascularization strategy will be eroded, providing a more even playing field.

Economic Impact of the Heart Team

There is currently no published data on the economic impact of revascularization heart teams, especially as the benefits are often intangible, e.g., the generation of research ideas, greater team satisfaction through collaboration, and greater patient satisfaction. Better patient outcomes influenced by the heart team decisions will only materialize in years to come. It would be expected that by determining the most appropriate revascularization strategy for patients based on evidence, long-term outcomes are improved and where CABG is avoided when inappropriate, length of stay in hospital is shortened, which would translate into cost savings in the healthcare system.

Conclusion

It is without doubt that attempting to change an ingrained culture of practice in well-established organizations is a daunting task. Fresh, foreign ideas are at times viewed with suspicion, and require a slow dismantling of supporting structures. A reliance on solid data to prove that outcomes can be altered by collaboration instead of competition, with delicate handling of egos, is the only way forward. Trials such as SYNTAX III make it exciting times for adopters of the heart team approach, but will no doubt face resistance from the traditional "gatekeepers."

"Little strokes fell great oaks."

References

1. Patel MR, Calhoon JH, Dehmer GJ, Grantham JA, Maddox TM, Maron DJ, et al. ACC/AATS/AHA/ASE/ASNC/SCAI/SCCT/STS 2017 appropriate use criteria for coronary revascularization in patients with stable ischemic heart disease: a report of the American College of Cardiology Appropriate Use Criteria Task Force, American Association for Thoracic Surgery, American Heart Association, American Society of Echocardiography, American Society of Nuclear Cardiology, Society for Cardiovascular Angiography and Interventions, Society of Cardiovascular Computed Tomography, and Society of Thoracic Surgeons. J Am Coll Cardiol. 2017;69(17):2212–41.

2. Neumann FJ, Sousa-Uva M, Ahlsson A, Alfonso F, Banning AP, Benedetto U, et al. 2018 ESC/EACTS guidelines on myocardial revascularization. Eur Heart J. 2019;40(2):87–165.
3. Schwalm JD, Wijeysundera HC, Tu JV, Guo H, Kingsbury KJ, Natarajan MK. Influence of coronary anatomy and SYNTAX score on the variations in revascularization strategies for patients with multivessel disease. Can J Cardiol. 2014;30(10):1155–61.
4. Toyota T, Morimoto T, Shiomi H, Ando K, Ono K, Shizuta S, et al. Ad hoc vs. non-ad hoc percutaneous coronary intervention strategies in patients with stable coronary artery disease. Circ J. 2017;81(4):458–67.
5. Hannan EL, Racz MJ, Gold J, Cozzens K, Stamato NJ, Powell T, et al. Adherence of catheterization laboratory cardiologists to American College of Cardiology/American Heart Association guidelines for percutaneous coronary interventions and coronary artery bypass graft surgery: what happens in actual practice? Circulation. 2010;121(2):267–75.
6. Sianos G, Morel MA, Kappetein AP, Morice MC, Colombo A, Dawkins K, et al. The SYNTAX score: an angiographic tool grading the complexity of coronary artery disease. EuroIntervention. 2005;1(2):219–27.
7. Garot P, Tafflet M, Kumar S, Salvatella N, Darremont O, Jouven X, et al. Reproducibility and factors influencing the assessment of the SYNTAX score in the left main Xience study. Catheter Cardiovasc Interv. 2012;80(2):231–7.
8. Genereux P, Palmerini T, Caixeta A, Cristea E, Mehran R, Sanchez R, et al. SYNTAX score reproducibility and variability between interventional cardiologists, core laboratory technicians, and quantitative coronary measurements. Circ Cardiovasc Interv. 2011;4(6):553–61.
9. Tanboga IH, Ekinci M, Isik T, Kurt M, Kaya A, Sevimli S. Reproducibility of syntax score: from core lab to real world. J Interv Cardiol. 2011;24(4):302–6.
10. Shiomi H, Tamura T, Niki S, Tada T, Tazaki J, Toma M, et al. Inter- and intra-observer variability for assessment of the synergy between percutaneous coronary intervention with TAXUS and cardiac surgery (SYNTAX) score and association of the SYNTAX score with clinical outcome in patients undergoing unprotected left main stenting in the real world. Circ J. 2011;75(5):1130–7.
11. Garg S, Girasis C, Sarno G, Goedhart D, Morel MA, Garcia-Garcia HM, et al. The SYNTAX score revisited: a reassessment of the SYNTAX score reproducibility. Catheter Cardiovasc Interv. 2010;75(6):946–52.
12. Banning AP, Baumbach A, Blackman D, Curzen N, Devadathan S, Fraser D, et al. Percutaneous coronary intervention in the UK: recommendations for good practice 2015. Heart. 2015;101(Suppl 3):1–13.
13. Al-Lamee R, Thompson D, Dehbi HM, Sen S, Tang K, Davies J, et al. Percutaneous coronary intervention in stable angina (ORBITA): a double-blind, randomised controlled trial. Lancet. 2018;391(10115):31–40.
14. Denvir MA, Pell JP, Lee AJ, Rysdale J, Prescott RJ, Eteiba H, et al. Variations in clinical decision-making between cardiologists and cardiac surgeons; a case for management by multidisciplinary teams? J Cardiothorac Surg. 2006;1:2.
15. Long J, Luckraz H, Thekkudan J, Maher A, Norell M. Heart team discussion in managing patients with coronary artery disease: outcome and reproducibility. Interact Cardiovasc Thorac Surg. 2012;14(5):594–8.
16. Pavlidis AN, Perera D, Karamasis GV, Bapat V, Young C, Clapp BR, et al. Implementation and consistency of heart team decision-making in complex coronary revascularisation. Int J Cardiol. 2016;206:37–41.
17. Brener SJ, Alapati V, Chan D, Da-Wariboko A, Kaid Y, Latyshev Y, et al. The SYNTAX II score predicts mortality at 4 years in patients undergoing percutaneous coronary intervention. J Invasive Cardiol. 2018;30(8):290–4.
18. Escaned J, Banning A, Farooq V, Echavarria-Pinto M, Onuma Y, Ryan N, et al. Rationale and design of the SYNTAX II trial evaluating the short to long-term outcomes of state-of-the-art percutaneous coronary revascularisation in patients with de novo three-vessel disease. EuroIntervention. 2016;12(2):e224–34.

19. Escaned J, Collet C, Ryan N, De Maria GL, Walsh S, Sabate M, et al. Clinical outcomes of state-of-the-art percutaneous coronary revascularization in patients with de novo three vessel disease: 1-year results of the SYNTAX II study. Eur Heart J. 2017;38(42):3124–34.
20. Modolo R, Collet C, Onuma Y, Serruys PW. SYNTAX II and SYNTAX III trials: what is the take home message for surgeons? Ann Cardiothorac Surg. 2018;7(4):470–82.
21. Cavalcante R, Onuma Y, Sotomi Y, Collet C, Thomsen B, Rogers C, et al. Non-invasive heart team assessment of multivessel coronary disease with coronary computed tomography angiography based on SYNTAX score II treatment recommendations: design and rationale of the randomised SYNTAX III revolution trial. EuroIntervention. 2017;12(16):2001–8.

Heart Teams for Aortic Valve Disease: The TAVI Revolution

3

Talal Al-Atassi and Marino Labinaz

Introduction

The prevalence of aortic valve stenosis (AS) has recently become clearer with previous hospital-based studies underestimating this disease burden. Within a population of 2500 patients older than 65 years followed in the community, the prevalence of mild and moderate-to-severe AS was 34.6% and 0.7%, respectively [1]. Given that the prevalence of AS increases exponentially with age and 8.3% of the North American population is predicted to be older than 75 years by 2025, the burden of AS will only continue to rise in the foreseeable future [2, 3]. This growing burden represents a major challenge at both the healthcare and hospital levels.

Patients with severe AS have a limited life expectancy if left to medical management [4]. The therapeutic options include surgical aortic valve replacement (SAVR) and, more recently, transcatheter aortic valve implantation (TAVI). Although inoperable patients previously did not have any viable options, TAVI is now an effective option to these patients, with proven superiority over medical therapy [5]. Recently, TAVI has been shown to be non-inferior to SAVR in high-risk [6, 7] and intermediate-risk patients [8, 9] and is currently being investigated in low-risk patients.

With the increase in medical complexity of an aging population and the therapeutic options available, the application of a Heart Team approach has become a pillar in the care of patients with severe AS supported by recommendations from Canadian, American, and European societies [10–12]. Herein, we explore the

T. Al-Atassi (✉)
University of Ottawa Heart Institute, Department of Surgery, Division of Cardiac Surgery, Ottawa, ON, Canada
e-mail: talatassi@ottawaheart.ca

M. Labinaz
University of Ottawa Heart Institute, Division of Cardiology, Ottawa, ON, Canada

© Springer Nature Switzerland AG 2019
T. Mesana (ed.), *Heart Teams for Treatment of Cardiovascular Disease*,
https://doi.org/10.1007/978-3-030-19124-5_3

history, composition, role, benefits, challenges, and future of the Heart Team evaluating AS in general, with specific anecdotes as it applies to the authors' center: The University of Ottawa Heart Institute (UOHI) in Ottawa, Canada.

History of the Heart Team

Multidisciplinary teams composed of various healthcare members working together to care for complex patients facing multiple therapeutic choices often spanning several medical and surgical specialties have a long history in the oncology and advanced heart failure fields. In the oncology world, the multidisciplinary cancer conference, also called the tumor board conference, has shown benefits in measurable outcomes including timeliness of treatment, continuity of care, and communication with referring clinicians, collection of data for research, adherence to clinical guidelines, effective resource utilization, improvement in workplace satisfaction through opportunities for professional development, and, in some cases, improved survival [13–16]. Data on improved survival through the use of multidisciplinary teams exists for colorectal, esophageal, head and neck, and breast cancer [13–16]. Similarly, multidisciplinary teams managing complex heart failure patients have decreased hospital readmissions and length of stay with improved patient quality of life and satisfaction [17–19].

The Heart Team in the contemporary sense originates from two randomized trials comparing surgical and percutaneous strategies in treating coronary disease and AS. Namely, these were the SYNTAX (Synergy Between PCI with Taxus and Cardiac Surgery) [20] and PARTNER (Placement of Aortic Transcatheter Valves) trials [5, 7]. In these trials, a Heart Team was used for selection of appropriate trial patients during screening. The Heart Team was initially composed of an interventional cardiologist and a cardiovascular surgeon. However, the definition of Heart Team was broadened by the American Centers for Medicare and Medicaid Services within the National Coverage Determination to embody collaboration and dedication across medical specialties to offer optimal patient-centered care, suggesting the addition of echocardiographers, imaging specialists, cardiac anesthesiologists, intensivists, nurses, and social workers.

TAVI Heart Team Mandate

The main objective of the TAVI Heart Team at The University of Ottawa Heart Institute (UOHI) is to facilitate timely access to safe and high-quality care for patients with aortic stenosis who are inoperable, or high-risk surgical candidates. As new data accumulates, the mandate of the Heart Team will likely expand to include all patients with symptomatic severe aortic stenosis. The Heart Team meets weekly to review patients referred for TAVI consideration. Members collaborate in decision-making around best options for patient care following contemporary guidelines. Occasionally, innovative and creative solutions must be applied in nonconventional

patients with AS for whom there are no guideline recommendations. The Heart Team manages referral volume and triages wait times to avoid delays in access to care within the constraints of a public healthcare system. For example, in-hospital patients admitted with congestive heart failure or patients with decreased left ventricular ejection fraction (LVEF) might be prioritized over stable, slightly symptomatic patients with preserved LVEF. Moreover, the Heart Team facilitates credible program development and addresses operational and practice issues as they arise, such as transitioning TAVIs from general anesthesia with endotracheal intubation to conscious sedation without intubation in the majority of patients. Another example is starting the first Canadian transcaval TAVI program, which provides a fully percutaneous alternative to transfemoral (TF) TAVI in patients with severe peripheral arterial disease who are not candidates for TF TAVI.

In parallel to the clinical roles, the TAVI Heart Team engages in local quality and research projects and commits to involvement in important multicenter trials, which ultimately help guide clinical practice. The Heart Team is also heavily involved in educating patients and their families and furnishing accurate educational resources. Finally, the Heart Team weekly meeting acts as an educational hub for medical students, residents, and fellows.

TAVI Heart Team Composition

Although the TAVI Heart Team originating from the PARTNER trial focused on the collaborative work between an interventional cardiologist and a surgeon, it has taken a much broader composition in real life clinical practice. Currently, the TAVI Heart Team at the UOHI is composed of the following members:

- Interventional cardiologists
- Cardiac surgeons
- Anesthesiologists
- Echocardiographers
- Radiologists
- Geriatricians
- Nurses (including operating room and catheterization lab managers as well as advanced practice nurses assuming the roles of coordinators and educators)

The presence of cardiac surgeons and interventional cardiologists is perhaps obvious, as it traces back to the original definition of the Heart Team in both research trials and practice. These two members build a collaborative partnership that not only provides complementary cognitive and technical expertise but also one that provides didactic, clinical, and ethical leadership in the understanding, adoption, and progression of TAVI, among traditional treatments for severe AS. Similar to many cardiac interventions, TAVI comes with its inherent risks, occasionally leading to death or major morbidity. Therefore, perceptions of biased or careless allocation can be detrimental to the patient, their family, and the institution. Hence, it is

important that TAVI is offered judiciously according to currently approved guidelines when it likely benefits the patient, and not because it exists as an alternative to surgery or based on economic considerations. We have found that the involvement of a cardiologist–surgeon team in screening, working up, performing implants, and managing TAVI patients has proved invaluable. Such a team brings credibility to the TAVI program, provides better clinical and technical preparedness for possible complications, and allows for greater acceptability should an unfavorable outcome occur due to shared decision-making. For example, we have insisted that the primary and secondary operator roles be alternated during TAVI implants. This applies to both the role of the cardiac surgeon during fully percutaneous transfemoral implant, as well as to the role of the interventional cardiologist during non-percutaneous TAVI. Alternating between the primary and secondary operator roles makes each operator facile at various procedural steps while gaining valuable pearls and mitigating pitfalls. Indeed, the cardiologists and surgeons bring different but complementary skill sets. The cardiologist's background involves more experience and facility with wires, fluoroscopic imaging, and percutaneous interventions, while a surgeon's background involves intimate knowledge of aortic root anatomy, intracardiac structures and relationships, and open vascular approaches. Toward the end of the learning curve, each member of a given team will have become competent both as a primary and secondary operator, and many a priori skills and knowledge differences may have disappeared and evolved into a new enhanced, hybrid operator. Furthermore, it is this collaborative relationship that allows for safe program development such as starting a percutaneous transcaval program or transitioning to a percutaneous transaxillary artery TAVI.

The anesthesiologists play a pivotal role within our TAVI Heart Team. They provide important recommendations for preoperative optimization, and they have been instrumental in the safe transition from TAVI done under general anesthesia with endotracheal intubation to conscious sedation without intubation in the majority of patients. This has led to improved outcomes and shorter lengths of stay. Anesthesiologists provide continuous intraoperative monitoring, and occasionally transesophageal echocardiography guidance, in complex cases done under general anesthesia. Postoperatively, anesthesiologists provide intensive care management for a subset of our TAVI patients with surgical access.

Echocardiographers with expertise in the aortic valve often provide further diagnostic guidance in complex borderline cases such as low-flow, low-gradient AS; symptomatic moderate AS; and asymptomatic severe AS. Similarly, their input is crucial in degenerated prosthetic valves, multivalvular pathology, and TAVI patients with sudden increase in gradients during follow-up. They also provide decisive intraoperative information during conscious sedation procedures. For example, they evaluate valve positioning and function right after deployment, assess for valvular regurgitation (trans- and paravalvular), and rule out any iatrogenic complications such as pericardial effusions and aortic complications.

Assessment for TAVI suitability often relies on anatomic factors, which is most accurately assessed using computed tomography (CT) scans. In the last 15 years, valve-sizing methods transitioned from echocardiographic-based aortic annular

measurements to using CT measurements of annular dimensions such as diameter, perimeter, and area, which proved more accurate and almost eliminated complications of valve embolization and annular rupture. Central to this assessment are radiologists experienced in CT scan assessments. The radiologists also provide information regarding valvular and subvalvular calcification, ascending aortic calcification, sinuses of Valsalva diameters, coronary heights, and assessment of vascular access including size, tortuosity, and calcification. Without accurate knowledge of all the above information, TAVI procedures would remain fraught with danger. Many complications can be averted using the information and measurements provided by radiologists at our weekly TAVI Heart Team meeting. In addition to data influencing the TAVI procedure, we often encounter incidental findings on CT scans. Radiologists can shed some light in regard to the necessity of further investigations and suspicion of malignancy in some cases. This information may influence the prognosis and projected survival in these patients, and can be an important determinant for the suitability of TAVI. Alternatively, a patient with an incidentally discovered malignancy with good prognosis and who is eligible for both SAVR and TAVI may be better treated with TAVI to expedite postoperative recovery and initiation of life-prolonging cancer treatment.

As the aging population continues to grow and their complexity continues to increase, decision-making in patients with AS will concordantly become more challenging. The presence of an expert geriatrician within the Heart Team helps us navigate through challenging cases by providing detailed assessments of patients' mental and physical reserves. This assessment of frailty is as important as assessing traditional predictors of mortality. In fact, there are reports that frailty may be more discriminative of 30-day mortality than the traditional Society of Thoracic Surgeons (STS) predicted risk of mortality [21].

Nurses by far have the closest interaction with patients. Their role within the Heart Team is multifactorial. The TAVI coordinator and the patient educator roles are assumed by advanced practice nurses, and they are often the backbone of the TAVI program. They facilitate a smooth transition through all phases of care and act as a liaison between the referring clinicians and the Heart Team, between various members of the Heart Team, and between the patient, their families, and the healthcare team. At our center, they help collate all patient information and manage our wait list. They also assist in ensuring patients move seamlessly through the healthcare system, which is particularly important for those patients with multiple medical issues. Finally, they ensure that accurate data is entered in our databases to enable research and assessment of outcomes. Operating room and catheterization lab nurse managers ensure readiness for procedures from an inventory, time, and nursing needs allocation on a certain day.

Benefits of TAVI Heart Team

The TAVI Heart Team potentially benefits many stakeholders in the healthcare system including the patients and their families, the healthcare workers, and the healthcare system itself. At face value, decision-making in a multidisciplinary team has

important advantages over solitary decision-making. As discussed above, medicine is becoming increasingly complex, with various therapeutic options in elderly patients with more comorbidities. This is exacerbated by limitations of the supportive evidence in specific subgroups of patients (e.g., risk scores such as the STS score not containing data on frailty, liver cirrhosis, or porcelain aortas). The combined expertise of a Heart Team provides for a more thorough and balanced appraisal of a specific case. However, unlike multidisciplinary decision-making in oncology and heart failure, there is a dearth of research and data on TAVI Heart Teams. There is ample opportunity for health services research to ascertain the benefit and explore the optimal care delivery model.

From the patient's perspective, there are numerous advantages of a Heart Team. Patients often have greater satisfaction with delivery of care with improved knowledge of their disease and therapeutic options. They are often reassured with the fact that their cases are discussed in a multidisciplinary setting and with their involvement in shared decision-making, which leads to reduced decisional conflict.

From the clinician's perspective, the Heart Team provides a platform for expanding clinical and procedural skill sets and allows for shared responsibility of the outcome, with reduced decisional conflict. In complex cases lacking support from protocols and guidelines, creative and innovative solutions can often be born during Heart Team discussions, with the opportunity to share responsibility for these novel treatments or strategies. In most instances, there is improved workplace satisfaction by being involved in a Heart Team, unless there is a toxic relationship between members of the Heart Team, which can sometimes undermine this advantage. However, by working together, the traditional competitive relationship between surgeons and cardiologists has changed into a more collaborative and collegial one. Furthermore, the Heart Team meetings can be instrumental to the education of medical students, residents, and fellows in one of the most rapidly evolving arenas in medicine.

At the healthcare system level, the advantages of a Heart Team include reduction in variability both in access and outcome. By ensuring greater adherence to guidelines and an unbiased and balanced appraisal, Heart Teams can minimize overutilization of an expensive therapeutic modality in patients who may not benefit from TAVI, while reducing underutilization of this life-saving therapy in inoperable and high-risk patients who may not otherwise have been referred. The TAVI Heart Team standardizes preoperative diagnostic work-ups, decreases time to decision, improves coordination and communication of care, shortens length of stay, and decreases readmission rates, all of which are cost-lowering strategies for the healthcare system.

TAVI Heart Team Challenges and Barriers

Despite all the discussed benefits of a TAVI Heart Team, there remain some important challenges and barriers that prevent it from operating at full potential. First, Heart Team meetings are time-consuming and difficult to organize. An increasing number of TAVI procedures and AS referrals means that the Heart Team meeting in

its current weekly form will become insufficient to adequately discuss all patients and fulfill its mandate as discussed above. Furthermore, as centers of excellence mature with regard to the knowledge base needed for patient evaluation, there may be less need for detailed review and planning by the whole Heart Team in its weekly meeting for straightforward cases. Moreover, as we embark on treating intermediate- and perhaps low-risk patients who have two viable treatment options, current Heart Team weekly meetings do not respond to the call in the most recent valve guidelines recommending that Heart Teams ensure that patient "expectations can be met as fully as possible using a shared decision-making approach." Answering such a call would involve a dedicated "Heart Valve Clinic" where the discussion and decision takes place with the patient, as will be discussed in a subsequent section, "Future of TAVI Heart Teams." Second, it is highly inefficient for physicians to participate in such Heart Teams based on existing payment mechanisms. The root cause for this is that time spent on procedures continues to be rewarded more than cognitive efforts. Although participation in Heart Teams could be seen as an opportunity to enlarge a center's referral base, it is difficult to see how a cardiac surgeon or interventional cardiologist would justify time away from the operating room or catheterization lab or why an echocardiographer, radiologist, or geriatrician would consistently attend such a meeting in the long-term. Without payers and policy makers tackling reimbursement head-on by incentivizing Heart Team meetings—as is done in the Netherlands—or for other Heart Teams within the UOHI such as heart failure, then meetings risk becoming a perfunctory process without true, integrated decision-making. This will lead to poor engagement, physician (and eventually patient) dissatisfaction, thus leading to poor outcomes. Third, without external evaluation or comparison with other centers' Heart Teams and TAVI programs, there is a risk of reinforcing prior biases when the same members continue to participate in Heart Team meetings. This can be mitigated by periodic external objective assessments of the Heart Team processes and outcomes. Furthermore, discussions with other center's Heart Teams can help share solutions to common challenges. Fourth, a lack of a central TAVI database within the institution, which can be easily linked to other programs, is a barrier to research and innovation. Ideally, every center would collect data on all AS patients in a similar format within an institutional database, which can be used for local research project. When required, the data from several institutions would be easily pooled for multicenter research projects. Alternatively, a provincial or national database can be created with institutional subdivisions, which would serve the same purpose. Although it can be seen as a large task in its initial stages, there are surely many potential rewards in terms of research and quality projects.

TAVI Heart Team Evaluation

In the era of evidence-based medicine, obtaining data is paramount to ensuring continued success of the TAVI Heart Team, while finding opportunities for growth and improvement. There are two ways in which the UOHI TAVI Heart Team

currently measures success. First, we collect data on a yearly basis and compare our progress longitudinally over time. Second, we compare the same data with other institutions in the province as well as with the most current published literature as a form of cross-sectional comparison. The collected data reflects both process and outcome measures of the TAVI program. Some of the metrics evaluating process include the number of monthly referrals and wait times; number of TAVIs performed on each TAVI day, monthly, and in the fiscal year; number of cancellations and reasons for these cancellations; and hospital lengths of stay. For example, in the last year, we transitioned from general anesthesia to conscious sedation in almost all of our transfemoral access TAVIs. This allowed our hospital length of stay to decrease from 10 days to 6 days. We also transitioned from routine two-transfemoral TAVI days to routine three-transfemoral TAVI days, with one proof-of-concept day when we performed four transfemoral TAVIs. Increasing efficiency allowed our average monthly wait times to drop from around 75 days to around 40 days. Finally, from a programmatic point of view, we began the first Canadian Transcaval access TAVI with 17 cases done to date, with excellent outcomes.

In addition to process, we collect outcome measures that include characteristics of our patients (acuity, STS score, etc), mortality, stroke and myocardial infarction at 30 days, minor and major vascular complications, permanent pacemaker insertion rate, hospital length of stay, and 30-day readmission rates. This data is compared with other institutions and with published data in the literature, which should identify potential gaps and opportunities for growth and improvement. For example, despite decreasing our hospital length of stay from 10 to 6 days, this still remains higher than many other institutions. This has led to a revamp of our post-TAVI protocols and education tools to allow for safe discharge when possible. We are also in the process of introducing and implementing the "Vancouver 3-M Clinical Pathway," which has shown safe 24–48-hour discharge [22].

The Future of TAVI Heart Team

With a growing population of elderly patients with AS and multiple other comorbidities coupled with the broadening of TAVI indications, there will certainly be more pressure on the TAVI Heart Team. The current form of weekly TAVI meetings will not be sustainable for timely access and decision-making for all of these patients. Although the waiting time between decision and procedure decreased significantly in the last year, there remain significant delays between referral, testing, meeting the interventional cardiologist or surgeon, and discussion at the multidisciplinary meeting. The future of the TAVI Heart Team will be within the context of a "Heart Valve Clinic" in an expert "Heart Valve Center," as demonstrated in Fig. 3.1.

Any patient who is diagnosed with AS should be referred to a Heart Valve Clinic within a Heart Valve Center, defined as a center with expertise in all facets of heart valve disease including diagnosis and interventions (percutaneous and surgical). Expertise in this case would entail high volume of all valve interventions with excellent outcomes. Participants in the Heart Valve Clinic would include a cardiac

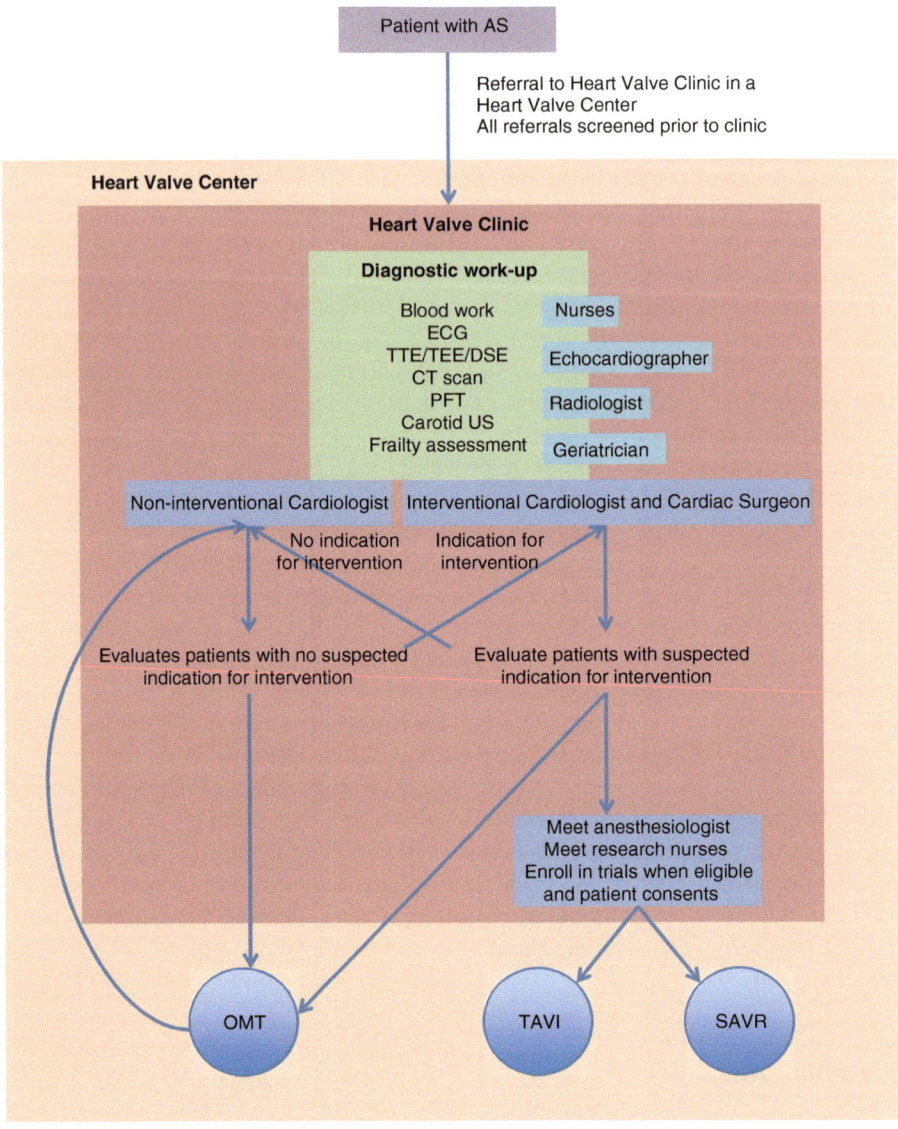

Fig. 3.1 Proposed future model of patient flow in a Heart Valve Clinic within a Heart Valve Center. AS, aortic stenosis; ECG, electrocardiogram; TTE, transthoracic echocardiogram; TEE, transesophageal echocardiogram; DSE, dobutamine stress echocardiogram; PFT, pulmonary function test; US, ultrasound; OMT, optimal medical therapy; TAVI, transcatheter aortic valve implantation; SAVR, surgical aortic valve replacement

surgeon, an interventional cardiologist, a non-interventional cardiologist, an anesthesiologist, a geriatrician, a radiologist, nurses, and program coordinators (including research nurses and coordinators).

The patients to be seen in such a clinic would be prescreened from the charts ahead of time to plan for the institutional capacity of diagnostic tests on that particular clinic day. The non-interventional cardiologist would see patients who are not ready for intervention from the initial chart screen. The interventional cardiologist and surgeon would see all patients who may meet an indication for intervention. The patients receive all diagnostic work-up, not already performed, in the same visit. This includes transthoracic or transesophageal echocardiograms, dobutamine stress echocardiograms, CT scans, pulmonary function tests, carotid ultrasounds, electrocardiograms, and blood work. The only exception would be procedures that require contrast (CT scan and coronary angiograms), which may have to be spaced several days apart. In that case, a coronary angiogram would be done prior to this clinic visit and the CT would be done on the day of the clinic. The geriatrician would assess appropriate patients for frailty. All cases would then be discussed in the clinic along with the patients and their families to ensure shared decision-making. The decision would take place for the vast majority of patients on that same day. Those patients that require additional investigations or more detailed discussion would be brought to the Heart Team meeting. The overall Heart Team would also provide oversight on the activities of the clinic to ensure best-practice guidelines are followed. This may be in the form of circulating the decisions made for clinic patients to all members of the Heart Team to be "signed off" on a weekly basis. The patient would then meet the anesthesiologist in the same clinic and a tentative date for the procedure would be offered before the patient leaves the clinic. Patients who may be eligible for inclusion into research trials will be screened, approached, and consented in the same clinic. Any admitted in-patients would be discussed on that same day as part of the multidisciplinary clinic as well. This Heart Valve Clinic framework would target several objectives simultaneously. It ensures efficient diagnostic work-up, timely and shared decision-making, timely and appropriate intervention for certain patients, and optimal medical therapy or appropriate expert follow-up for patients without an indication for intervention. The described model would apply to all valve disease, not only AS.

Conclusion

Although a multidisciplinary team approach to cancers and heart failure is well established, the concept of a formal, multidisciplinary Heart Team in the areas of coronary revascularization and valve intervention is a more recent development. It was born within a research trial context and soon became the standard that is recommended by major Canadian, American, and European societies and guidelines. It has provided a hub for discussing complex patients and reaching unbiased decisions in an efficient manner. However, with increased TAVI volume, the Heart Team will likely take on a different form in the near future to keep its efficiency, while involving the patient within the decision-making process. This form will likely be as a Heart Valve Clinic within a Heart Valve Center.

References

1. d'Arcy JL, Coffey S, Loudon MA, Kennedy A, Pearson-Stuttard J, Birks J, et al. Large-scale community echocardiographic screening reveals a major burden of undiagnosed valvular heart disease in older people: the OxVALVE Population Cohort Study. Eur Heart J. 2016;37(47):3515–22.
2. Eveborn GW, Schirmer H, Heggelund G, Lunde P, Rasmussen K. The evolving epidemiology of valvular aortic stenosis. The Tromso study. Heart. 2013;99(6):396–400.
3. Osnabrugge RL, Mylotte D, Head SJ, Van Mieghem NM, Nkomo VT, LeReun CM, et al. Aortic stenosis in the elderly: disease prevalence and number of candidates for transcatheter aortic valve replacement: a meta-analysis and modeling study. J Am Coll Cardiol. 2013;62(11):1002–12.
4. Clark MA, Arnold SV, Duhay FG, Thompson AK, Keyes MJ, Svensson LG, et al. Five-year clinical and economic outcomes among patients with medically managed severe aortic stenosis: results from a Medicare claims analysis. Circ Cardiovasc Qual Outcomes. 2012;5(5):697–704.
5. Leon MB, Smith CR, Mack M, Miller DC, Moses JW, Svensson LG, et al. Transcatheter aortic-valve implantation for aortic stenosis in patients who cannot undergo surgery. N Engl J Med. 2010;363(17):1597–607.
6. Adams DH, Popma JJ, Reardon MJ, Yakubov SJ, Coselli JS, Deeb GM, et al. Transcatheter aortic-valve replacement with a self-expanding prosthesis. N Engl J Med. 2014;370(19):1790–8.
7. Smith CR, Leon MB, Mack MJ, Miller DC, Moses JW, Svensson LG, et al. Transcatheter versus surgical aortic-valve replacement in high-risk patients. N Engl J Med. 2011;364(23):2187–98.
8. Leon MB, Smith CR, Mack MJ, Makkar RR, Svensson LG, Kodali SK, et al. Transcatheter or surgical aortic-valve replacement in intermediate-risk patients. N Engl J Med. 2016;374(17):1609–20.
9. Reardon MJ, Van Mieghem NM, Popma JJ, Kleiman NS, Søndergaard L, Mumtaz M, et al. Surgical or transcatheter aortic-valve replacement in intermediate-risk patients. N Engl J Med. 2017;376(14):1321–31.
10. Nishimura RA, Otto CM, Bonow RO, Carabello BA, Erwin JP 3rd, Guyton RA, et al. 2014 AHA/ACC guideline for the management of patients with valvular heart disease: a report of the American College of Cardiology/American Heart Association task force on practice guidelines. J Thorac Cardiovasc Surg. 2014;148(1):e1–e132.
11. Vahanian A, Alfieri O, Andreotti F, Antunes MJ, Barón-Esquivias G, Baumgartner H, et al. Guidelines on the management of valvular heart disease (version 2012): the joint task force on the management of valvular heart disease of the European Society of Cardiology (ESC) and the European Association for Cardio-Thoracic Surgery (EACTS). Eur J Cardiothorac Surg. 2012;42(4):S1–44.
12. Webb J, Rodés-Cabau J, Fremes S, Pibarot P, Ruel M, Ibrahim R, et al. Transcatheter aortic valve implantation: a Canadian Cardiovascular Society position statement. Can J Cardiol. 2012;28(5):520–8.
13. Croke JM, El-Sayed S. Multidisciplinary management of cancer patients: chasing a shadow or real value? An overview of the literature. Curr Oncol. 2012;19(4):e232–8.
14. Freeman RK, Van Woerkom JM, Vyverberg A, Ascioti AJ. The effect of a multidisciplinary thoracic malignancy conference on the treatment of patients with lung cancer. Eur J Cardiothorac Surg. 2010;38(1):1–5.
15. Kesson EM, Allardice GM, George WD, Burns HJ, Morrison DS. Effects of multidisciplinary team working on breast cancer survival: retrospective, comparative, interventional cohort study of 13,722 women. BMJ. 2012;344:e2718.
16. Taylor C, Munro AJ, Glynne-Jones R, Griffith C, Trevatt P, Richards M, et al. Multidisciplinary team working in cancer: what is the evidence? BMJ. 2010;340:c951.
17. Del Sindaco D, Pulignano G, Minardi G, Apostoli A, Guerrieri L, Rotoloni M, et al. Two-year outcome of a prospective, controlled study of a disease management programme for elderly patients with heart failure. J Cardiovasc Med (Hagerstown). 2007;8(5):324–9.

18. Ducharme A, Doyon O, White M, Rouleau JL, Brophy JM. Impact of care at a multidisciplinary congestive heart failure clinic: a randomized trial. CMAJ. 2005;173(1):40–5.
19. Takeda A, Taylor SJ, Taylor RS, Khan F, Krum H, Underwood M. Clinical service organisation for heart failure. Cochrane Database Syst Rev. 2012;(9):CD002752.
20. Serruys PW, Morice MC, Kappetein AP, Colombo A, Holmes DR, Mack MJ, et al. Percutaneous coronary intervention versus coronary-artery bypass grafting for severe coronary artery disease. N Engl J Med. 2009;360(10):961–72.
21. Forcillo J, Condado JF, Ko YA, Yuan M, Binongo JN, Ndubisi NM, et al. Assessment of commonly used frailty markers for high- and extreme-risk patients undergoing transcatheter aortic valve replacement. Ann Thorac Surg. 2017;104(6):1939–46.
22. Lauck SB, Wood DA, Baumbusch J, Kwon JY, Stub D, Achtem L, et al. Vancouver transcatheter aortic valve replacement clinical pathway: minimalist approach, standardized care, and discharge criteria to reduce length of stay. Circ Cardiovasc Qual Outcomes. 2016;9(3):312–21.

The Mitral Valve Heart Team

4

David Messika-Zeitoun, Anthony Tran, Benjamin Hibbert, and Vincent Chan

Introduction

Mitral valve (MV) disease is a leading disease cause of mortality and morbidity in Western countries. Moderate or severe MV diseases are notably common in the community—in fact as common aortic valve diseases—and prevalence of MV disease increases with age. Thus, the reported prevalence of MV disease is 1.7% in the general population, increasing to up to 9% in those above 75 years [1]. With the aging of the population, prevalence of MV disease is expected to even further markedly increase, and MV disease should be considered as an important public-health problem.

Although the generic reasons for implementing a MV heart team (HT) are grossly not different than those from the other cardiac fields, the complexity and heterogeneity of MV diseases, the current unmet medical need, as well as the critical expertise required to achieve the most optimal patient care deserve a special mention. These critical notions are illustrated in the two following vignette cases.

The first patient is an 82-year-old woman with a medical history of Parkinson's disease, diabetes, and moderate chronic kidney dysfunction. She was known for several years for mitral valve prolapse and severe mitral regurgitation. Eighteen

D. Messika-Zeitoun (✉)
Division of Cardiology, University of Ottawa Heart Institute, Ottawa, ON, Canada
e-mail: DMessika-zeitoun@ottawaheart.ca

A. Tran
University of Connecticut Health, Department of Surgery, Farmington, CT, USA
e-mail: antran@uchc.edu

B. Hibbert
Department of Medicine, Division of Cardiology, University of Ottawa Heart Institute, Ottawa, ON, Canada

V. Chan
Department of Surgery, University of Ottawa Heart Institute, Ottawa, ON, Canada

© Springer Nature Switzerland AG 2019
T. Mesana (ed.), *Heart Teams for Treatment of Cardiovascular Disease*,
https://doi.org/10.1007/978-3-030-19124-5_4

months ago, she suffered from a minor stroke when she started presenting episodes of atrial fibrillation. She was seen by a community cardiologist; a conservative management was advocated, as left ventricular ejection fraction (LVEF) was preserved and surgery was deemed at high risk. She remained stable for 12 months before complaining of worsening dyspnea and was recently admitted for congestive heart failure and transferred to our center for further evaluation. Last transthoracic echocardiography showed a reduced LVEF (40%), severely enlarged left atrium, and elevated right ventricular pressure. This case illustrates several major points, namely (1) insufficient knowledge regarding indications for interventions; (2) incorrect estimation of the risk/benefit ratio; (3) unduly delayed/denied intervention; and (4) the absence of referral to an expert team.

The second case is a 65-year-old man with a remote large inferior and lateral myocardial infarction 4 years ago. He presented late, and revascularization was performed after H12. Despite optimal medical therapy, LVEF remained reduced (35%) and he progressively developed a moderate to severe secondary MR. He is in NYHA class III but presented several episodes of acute congestive heart failure. Last coronary angiogram showed patent prior stent and no other significant stenosis. He received contradictory advice regarding whether a MV intervention was appropriate. This case illustrates (1) the heterogeneity of MV disease spectrum and (2) the uncertainties of management of certain subset of patients with MV disease.

In the present chapter, we will focus on mitral valve regurgitation (MR) since mitral valve stenosis is rarely observed in Western countries due to the major decrease in the prevalence of rheumatic disease. We first present the main reasons that underlie the creation of a dedicated MV heart team, propose our vision of how the MV heart team should be implemented after highlighting the potential benefit and challenges it may face, and finally touch on how to monitor its efficiency both at the patient level and, more broadly, at the institutional and regional level.

Why Implement a Mitral Valve Heart Team?

A complex anatomy with multiple mechanisms and etiologies is a TITLE as a challenging echo. The mitral valve apparatus is composed of two leaflets attached through chordae to the anterolateral and posterolateral papillary muscles. Both leaflets are attached to the mitral annulus. Abnormality in any of these components, leaflets, chordae, annulus, papillary muscle, and adjacent myocardium can lead to a MV dysfunction causing MR. It is critical to differentiate primary MR, which refers to direct lesion of the valve/chordae, from secondary MR, in which functional incompetence of a valve otherwise anatomically normal is due to regional LV remodelling. Secondary MR occurs mainly in the setting of ischemic heart disease or dilated cardiomyopathy. This subdivision is not purely formal or academic, but has profound implication regarding both patients' evaluation and management [2–4].

A Challenging Echocardiographic Evaluation

Echocardiography (both transthoracic and transesophageal) is the mainstay of the evaluation of patients with MV disease. Echocardiography allows precise assessment of the mechanism and etiology of the regurgitation as well as an accurate evaluation of its severity. Recent advance in imaging, and more specifically of 3D echocardiography, has profoundly changed evaluation of MR etiology and mechanism as well as has allowed development—through accurate guidance— of transcatheter therapies [5]. A high-quality echocardiographic evaluation—requiring specific training and expertise not available in any center—including triple quantitation of left atrial size, LV size and function as well MR severity is of utmost importance [6]. Albeit not perfect and portending both limitations and pitfalls, the PISA method is probably the more widely available and useful method [7, 8]. Interestingly, detractors of the PISA do not provide any simple and robust alternative.

Multiplicity of Therapeutic Options: An Advocacy for Expert Reference Centers

In contrast to aortic valve stenosis, for which both etiologies and treatment are almost rigorously identical for all patients (aortic valve replacement using bio-prosthetic or mechanical valve for both degenerative bicuspid and tricuspid aortic valve stenosis), a tailored "a la carte" approach correcting each specific lesion can be proposed for MR [9]. It is now well established that MV repair is the treatment of choice for primary MR and is associated with both better immediate- and long-term results than MV replacement [10, 11]. However, performance of MV repair—even after adjustment for patients' characteristics—markedly varied across countries, centers, and even among surgeons of the same institution [12, 13]. This heterogeneity has been alluded to as the "lottery of MV repair surgery." Concentration of MV surgery to regional reference centers capable of providing the full spectrum of MV corrections has been advocated in order to allow more equitable access to MV repair. This full spectrum encompasses mitral transcatheter therapies that are now also available [14–16] following the booming of transcatheter aortic valve replacement [17]. Uncertainties regarding optimal management of secondary MR either concomitantly at the time of coronary artery bypass grafting, in isolation during surgery (MV repair or replacement), or using transcatheter therapies add another level of complexity [18–22]. Use of the Mitraclip system® in patients with secondary MR is expected to significantly increase in the years to come, but the opposite results of the two recent randomized controlled trials require the identification of subsets of patients that may benefit from the procedure.

Major Gaps Between Recommendations of National and International Societies and Current Clinical Practice

For the first patient, an intervention was considered late in the course of the disease when she was severely symptomatic in atrial fibrillation with significant left ventricular dysfunction, which increases surgical risks and adversely impacts long-term survival despite the valvular intervention [23–26]. Optimal management of patients with MR requires (1) accurate screening for disease; (2) appropriate follow-up; and (3) timely intervention and individualized therapeutic decision. In addition to the underdiagnosis of valvular heart diseases, which is outside the scope of the present chapter, poor knowledge regarding appropriate management/current guidelines is a major reason for such gaps between recommendations and clinical practice. A recent community cohort study performed at the Mayo Clinic clearly demonstrates an undertreatment of patients with mitral regurgitation due to an insufficient knowledge. All patients had an echocardiography providing an accurate assessment of the severity of the disease that was transmitted to the treating physician, but despite presence of guideline-based class I surgical indications, only one-fifth of the population underwent a mitral valve surgery [27]. A survey performed in a wide range of European practitioners to assess both perceived needs in knowledge, skills, and confidence, and actual practice according to case scenarios, confirmed this insufficient knowledge in the appropriate management of patients with valvular heart disease (VHD) [28]. The first vignette also illustrates the incorrect assessment of the benefit/risk ratio by the community cardiologist, which is relatively common in the setting of MR. As for other disease, surgical-risk scores [29–32] are unperfect, requiring a more comprehensive evaluation including frailty and life-expectancy evaluation by dedicated healthcare specialists including surgeons, anesthesiologists, and geriatricians to perform more accurate risk-benefit assessment. Even more importantly, reasons advocated not to intervene are often inappropriate. In the Euro Heart Survey, the surgery was denied in half of patients with severe symptomatic MR; impaired LVEF, older age, and comorbidity were the most striking characteristics of patients who were denied surgery, with an excessive and unjustified weight of age and LVEF in the decision [33].

Implementation of the Mitral Valve Heart Team

A heart team is a multidisciplinary group of physicians and allied healthcare professionals combining their expertise in order to achieve the most optimal and tailored patient care, i.e., optimizing patient-centered care. The team members, experts in the field of the mitral valve, should be able to offer an integrated care and tackle all issues associated with patient management from patient's selection, risk assessment, and treatment decision to state-of-the-art performance of both surgical and transcatheter interventions and follow-up.

Potential Benefit of the MV Heart Team

One main benefit of the MV heart team is to implement a standardized process for both evaluation and management of patients with MV disease. Through a central and unique referral pattern, appropriate tests will be scheduled and performed before the patient's management will be discussed by the team. This centralization and the improvement of the referral pathways should lead, but not limited, to a decrease in waiting times.

A second important benefit is the collaborative and open decision regarding the patient's management. The MV team will carefully evaluate all available therapeutic options and select the most appropriate one for a given patient. Transparency of the decision markedly relieves an important bias relative to individual physician's preferences and expertise. Considering the scarcity of resources in most centers and countries, the MV heart team may also improve efficiency and cost-effectiveness by selecting the right treatment for the right patient and may act as a safeguard avoiding futile and costly interventions. At the same time, the heart team will provide adequate treatment to patients who could have been otherwise unduly denied any intervention, as shown in the Euro Heart Survey. The discussion of all therapeutic options and sharing the recommendation/opinion of the heart team with patients and their families also allows more informed and engaged patient decisions. Importantly, the diversity of background of the team members may prompt more specific focus on the patient's considerations and expectations rather than on those of an individual physician.

The heart team is a gathering health professionals who may have divergent views. Confrontation of these potentially divergent opinions to reach a common decision by all team members helps in the team building. The shared accountability of the decision is beneficial for both the patients and their families, but also to the physicians when a severe complication occurs, as in most cases the heart team is dealing with complex patients. The experience of sharing decisions, the habits to regularly meet and discuss therapeutic options, as well as performing the interventions together also markedly add to the team spirit building. It improves communication between members before, during, and after interventions. The implementation of a successful MV team is also expected to increase referral locally and more broadly. These successes also increase the visibility of the team, which may be given rapid access to new technologies.

The MV heart team also provides unique opportunities for training, education, and research. Medical students and residents who are integrated into the team will be exposed to a unique concentration of complex cases as well as to discussions of all—including novel—therapeutic options. Confrontation of opinions and discussions between team members also increases the knowledge of each team member and may create the opportunity for the development of new innovative and creative therapeutic solutions. The heart team is also ideally positioned to develop dedicated databases that could be analyzed locally or combined with those of similar MV heart teams.

Challenges

However, creation of a MV team is not an easy task, and several challenges should be taken into consideration. The first challenge is the paradigm shift from an individual solitary decision to a group and shared model decision. The patient is not referred to a single individual who will decide what is best for the patient, but the decision is made collectively. This is a profound cultural change that relies on acceptance by all team members of the final decision. Issues may arise when no consensus can be reached, and a process must be defined in advance to tackle this issue such as a vote or the final word given to the team leader. It is also critical to build trust between members regarding both their expertise and judgment, which takes time. Competition may nevertheless arise between team members. Unintentionally or not, surgeons may be more prone to offer a surgical option, whereas interventional cardiologists may be more prone to propose a transcatheter intervention. Such competition is further exemplified in a fee-for-service model where salary of the operator depends on numbers. The opportunity for the surgeons to also perform transcatheter MV intervention markedly clears out this type of concern.

The heart team may also face critical logistic issues, as both money and time are involved in the heart team building process and are scarce resources. It is often difficult to coordinate schedules and availability for team members to meet on a regular basis. In addition, in a fee-for-service model, time spent in meetings is not considered. Reimbursement of MV heart team meetings could be envisaged.

Another important drawback of the fee-for-service model is to limit the participation of echocardiographers to the procedure. This is critical, as they usually perform the screening evaluation (and follow-up) that may be disconnected from what the surgeon/interventional cardiologist are expecting, due to lack of expertise. Involvement of an echocardiographer as interventional echocardiographer guiding the procedure should be encouraged. A shared billing model between interventionalist and echocardiographers may allow the latter to participate in the procedure, which improves involvement, quality of the examination performed, and team spirit.

The heart team meetings may also induce some delay in decisions, which may be largely counterbalanced by the potential benefit of the MV heart team, but raises issues when more urgent decisions are needed, such as for inpatients. Use of new communication channels such as MV heart team group app represents an attractive solution. As mentioned above, centralization of the referral and standardization of the evaluation require a high level of care coordination. The role of the coordinator staff is in this regard critical, as he or she will oversee centralizing all referrals. This also will be a cultural change, especially in highly competitive and individualistic environments. This coordination is both time- and resource-consuming. Implementation of a MV heart team thus requires institutional resources (immediate cost of implementation of the HT). Despite all these challenges, TAVR heart team has been successfully implemented in the USA, where the fee-for-service model is highly competitive and business-driven.

The MV Heart Team in Practice

In this section we present our vision of the MV heart team, its composition, governance, and operational mode. The core of the team should be composed of at least one cardiac surgeon, one interventional cardiologist, one clinical cardiologist/echocardiographer, one heart failure specialist, one cardiac anesthesiologist, and one senior nursing coordinator. When needed, a rapid access to a geriatrician or to other specialists should be made available. One of the team members should take the leadership of the team and more closely work with the nurse coordinator. The team should meet on a weekly basis at a time suiting most members, and discuss all patients referred. Early morning is often the best timing. It is also critical to obtain and present the immediate- and mid-term outcomes of patients presented at the MV meeting whether a surgical, transcatheter, or conservative management has been advocated. Trust and confidence should be built during these meetings as well as during interventions.

The issue of referral raises several important questions: should all patients with MV disease be discussed, should the MV team be an isolated or integrated structure, and should the MV heart team be implemented in all centers? As discussed below, these questions are closely intricated. Referring all patients with MV disease to the MV heart team is time-consuming and not a realistic model. In addition, management of patients with primary MR is often straightforward. Class I and IIa indication for intervention has been clearly defined, and these patients will only marginally benefit from a heart team assessment that should be restricted to complex patients. In contrast, patients with severe primary MR symptomatic (or with other class I/IIa indication such as atrial fibrillation, elevated right ventricular systolic pressure, or reduced ejection fraction) and significant comorbidities should be discussed. Ideally, all patients with severe secondary MR should be discussed, especially when no coronary revascularization is needed. As mentioned previously, management of these patients remained debated with contradictory results. In our view, the MV team should be an emanation of the Valve Clinic [34]. In order to be adequately discussed at the MV heart team meeting, the patients should be referred to the Valve Clinic where a standardized comprehensive and extensive evaluation of the MV disease and comorbidities will be performed. More specifically, it is critical that the echocardiographer performing and reading the examination should be both dedicated and motivated in order to provide all the information to perform an informed decision including accurate quantitation of the regurgitation and of the MV disease mechanisms and lesions. In addition, in order to be adequately discussed and to take patient's wishes and expectations into consideration, the patient must be seen at the Valve Clinic by one of the team members. Informal discussions between the patient, family, and the nurse coordinator are also critical.

Implementation of the MV heart team should be restricted to Heart Valve Centers of Excellence. The center should provide the full armamentarium of MV surgical and transcatheter therapies, the team members should be experts in MV disease evaluation and management, and the surgeons be able to achieve high repair rates and low complications rates. Such results can only be obtained in high-volume

experienced centers in order to avoid the lottery of MV repair. Only MV teams implemented in such centers could expect to meet their mandate, i.e., achieving the most optimal state-of-the-art tailored patient care.

How to Monitor the Efficiency and Impact of the Mitral Valve Heart Team?

There are no reasons that the MV heart team will not provide similar benefits than the successful heart failure team, but proof/evidence of the benefit of MV team is currently limited. Evaluation of the efficiency of the MV heart team can be performed at multiple levels, from patient levels to institutional, provincial, or national levels, but there is a need to develop specific indicators.

The easiest parameters to monitor are probably those related to institutional processes. Several indicators can be proposed, such as the waiting time and the number of cases discussed by the MV heart team. Whether the MV heart team improves waiting time between referral and intervention is of interest. This waiting time could be subdivided as waiting time between referral and MV heart time decision and waiting time between MV heart time decision and intervention, this later being only partially under the control of the MV heart team. The centralized referral pathway as well as the standardized evaluation of MV disease, key elements the MV team should establish as mentioned above, are expected to decrease waiting times.

Number of cases discussed weekly by the MV heart team reflects, at least partially, the overall adoption rate of the MV heart team internally by the other colleagues, as well as externally by those of the surrounding area. It thus reflects the overall activity of the MV heart team and its changes over time. However, the absolute number of cases discussed may only reflect the increased incidence of MV disease. One important indicator would be the ratio of the number of cases discussed/overall number of similar cases seen at the level of the institution. Implementation of electronic medical records should facilitate identification of such cases, providing calculation of the denominator. Extension to the overall number of cases seen at the level of the entire surrounding area may be even more important, but requires a common shared electronic medical record with community hospitals and private clinics.

At an even broader level, one main indicator to establish would be the impact of the MV team on the appropriateness of care of patients with MV disease. It would require identification of all cases with severe MV disease and a class I or IIa indication for intervention according to current guidelines, assessment of comorbidities, and evaluation of, on one side, the rate of unduly denied/delayed intervention and, on the other side, the rate of appropriate conservative management (futile interventions).

Assessment of results is also critical, such as monitoring mortality and complication rates of the various MV interventions. However, such results are expected to be dependent of the case mix. Thus, with development of transcatheter therapies that are indicated to high-risk patients, a shift of the high-risk population from surgery toward transcatheter interventions is expected to be associated with an overall

decrease of the surgical mortality/complications rate that is unrelated to the MV heart team efficiency. Nevertheless, assessment of procedural success/complications rate of transcatheter therapies is an important information despite also depending on case mix. These rates could be compared across centers and countries. Higher rates would suggest selection of excessively high-risk patients or insufficient training. These rates could be adjusted to patients' profile and are important elements the MV heart team should collect. These indicators also raise the question of futility. What thresholds of immediate- and mid-term mortality are the institution and the stakeholders willing to accept and pay for? Calculation of incremental cost-effectiveness ratio (ICER) is important, and requires establishment of controls arms.

Finally, further to the evaluation of its efficiency, a cost-effectiveness evaluation of the implementation of the MV heart team should be performed. Such evaluation would rely on several of the indicators presented above and a careful follow-up of the patients, including readmission rates and disability. The question of whether the MV team—through the processes it has implemented and the quality and accuracy of its decisions—improves the cost-effectiveness of the management of complex patients with MV disease deserves to be evaluated.

Conclusion

The management of patients with mitral valve disease is becoming increasingly difficult due on one side the intrinsic complexity and heterogeneity of the disease, the uncertainties regarding the optimal management, the increasing rates of comorbidities, the technological advances and the expected the development of transcatheter therapies in the setting of both primary and secondary MR, and on the other side the significant gaps between current recommendations and effective management of patients with MV disease. Implementation of a mitral valve heart team gathering experts in the field of MV disease (surgeons, interventional cardiologists, echocardiographers, anesthesiologists and heart failure specialists) supported by a senior nurse coordinators staff to evaluate, manage and treat these patients is therefore critical.

These MV heart teams should be implemented and restricted to Heart Valve Centers of Excellence capable of providing the full armamentarium of MV therapies and excellent surgical/transcatheter outcomes. The MV heart team should be integrated as an emanation of the Valve Clinic, from which it will benefit from a standardized high-quality clinical and echocardiographic evaluation, and the MV heart team should specifically focus on complex/high-risk patients with both primary and secondary mitral regurgitation.

The mandate of the MV heart team is to provide the most optimal patient-centered care according to current evidence-based medicine. Its implementation is expected to provide marked benefit for both the patients and the institution, but also raises important challenges that should be addressed. It is therefore critical to monitor its efficiency and, more globally, its impact on the quality of care and its cost-effectiveness for the management of complex patients with MV disease.

References

1. Nkomo VT, Gardin JM, Skelton TN, Gottdiener JS, Scott CG, Enriquez-Sarano M. Burden of valvular heart diseases: a population-based study. Lancet. 2006;368(9540):1005–11.
2. Baumgartner H, Falk V, Bax JJ, De Bonis M, Hamm C, Holm PJ, et al. 2017 ESC/EACTS guidelines for the management of valvular heart disease. Eur Heart J. 2017;38(36):2739–91.
3. Nishimura RA, Otto CM, Bonow RO, Carabello BA, Erwin JP 3rd, Fleisher LA, et al. 2017 AHA/ACC focused update of the 2014 AHA/ACC guideline for the management of patients with valvular heart disease: a report of the American College of Cardiology/ American Heart Association task force on clinical practice guidelines. Circulation. 2017;135(25):e1159–95.
4. Nishimura RA, Otto CM, Bonow RO, Carabello BA, Erwin JP 3rd, Guyton RA, et al. 2014 AHA/ACC guideline for the management of patients with valvular heart disease: executive summary: a report of the American College of Cardiology/American Heart Association task force on practice guidelines. Circulation. 2014;129(23):2440–92.
5. Lang RM, Addetia K, Narang A, Mor-Avi V. 3-dimensional echocardiography: latest developments and future directions. JACC Cardiovasc Imaging. 2018;11(12):1854–78.
6. Zoghbi WA, Adams D, Bonow RO, Enriquez-Sarano M, Foster E, Grayburn PA, et al. Recommendations for noninvasive evaluation of native valvular regurgitation: a report from the American Society of Echocardiography developed in collaboration with the Society for Cardiovascular Magnetic Resonance. J Am Soc Echocardiogr. 2017;30(4):303–71.
7. Enriquez-Sarano M, Avierinos JF, Messika-Zeitoun D, Detaint D, Capps M, Nkomo V, et al. Quantitative determinants of the outcome of asymptomatic mitral regurgitation. N Engl J Med. 2005;352(9):875–83.
8. El-Tallawi KC, Messika-Zeitoun D, Zoghbi WA. Assessment of the severity of native mitral valve regurgitation. Prog Cardiovasc Dis. 2017;60(3):322–33.
9. Verma S, Mesana TG. Mitral-valve repair for mitral-valve prolapse. N Engl J Med. 2009;361(23):2261–9.
10. Braunberger E, Deloche A, Berrebi A, Abdallah F, Celestin JA, Meimoun P, et al. Very long-term results (more than 20 years) of valve repair with carpentier's techniques in nonrheumatic mitral valve insufficiency. Circulation. 2001;104(12 Suppl 1):I8–11.
11. Chan V, Ruel M, Chaudry S, Lambert S, Mesana TG. Clinical and echocardiographic outcomes after repair of mitral valve bileaflet prolapse due to myxomatous disease. J Thorac Cardiovasc Surg. 2012;143(4 Suppl):S8–11.
12. Chikwe J, Toyoda N, Anyanwu AC, Itagaki S, Egorova NN, Boateng P, et al. Relation of mitral valve surgery volume to repair rate, durability, and survival. J Am Coll Cardiol. 2017:pii:S0735-1097(17)30677-0.
13. Gammie JS, O'Brien SM, Griffith BP, Ferguson TB, Peterson ED. Influence of hospital procedural volume on care process and mortality for patients undergoing elective surgery for mitral regurgitation. Circulation. 2007;115(7):881–7.
14. Feldman T, Foster E, Glower DD, Kar S, Rinaldi MJ, Fail PS, et al. Percutaneous repair or surgery for mitral regurgitation. N Engl J Med. 2011;364(15):1395–406.
15. Messika-Zeitoun D, Nickenig G, Latib A, Kuck KH, Baldus S, Schueler R, et al. Transcatheter mitral valve repair for functional mitral regurgitation using the Cardioband system: 1 year outcomes. Eur Heart J. 2019;40(5):466–72.
16. Sorajja P, Mack M, Vemulapalli S, Holmes DR Jr, Stebbins A, Kar S, et al. Initial experience with commercial transcatheter mitral valve repair in the United States. J Am Coll Cardiol. 2016;67(10):1129–40.
17. Nguyen V, Michel M, Eltchaninoff H, Gilard M, Dindorf C, Iung B, et al. Implementation of transcatheter aortic valve replacement in France. J Am Coll Cardiol. 2018;71(15):1614–27.
18. Acker MA, Parides MK, Perrault LP, Moskowitz AJ, Gelijns AC, Voisine P, et al. Mitral-valve repair versus replacement for severe ischemic mitral regurgitation. N Engl J Med. 2013;370(1):23–32.

19. Goldstein D, Moskowitz AJ, Gelijns AC, Ailawadi G, Parides MK, Perrault LP, et al. Two-year outcomes of surgical treatment of severe ischemic mitral regurgitation. N Engl J Med. 2015;374(4):344–53.
20. Obadia JF, Messika-Zeitoun D, Leurent G, Iung B, Bonnet G, Piriou N, et al. Percutaneous repair or medical treatment for secondary mitral regurgitation. N Engl J Med. 2018;379(24):2297–306.
21. Smith PK, Puskas JD, Ascheim DD, Voisine P, Gelijns AC, Moskowitz AJ, et al. Surgical treatment of moderate ischemic mitral regurgitation. N Engl J Med. 2014;371(23):2178–88.
22. Stone GW, Lindenfeld J, Abraham WT, Kar S, Lim DS, Mishell JM, et al. Transcatheter mitral-valve repair in patients with heart failure. N Engl J Med. 2018;379(24):2307–18.
23. Barbieri A, Bursi F, Grigioni F, Tribouilloy C, Avierinos JF, Michelena HI, et al. Prognostic and therapeutic implications of pulmonary hypertension complicating degenerative mitral regurgitation due to flail leaflet: a multicenter long-term international study. Eur Heart J. 2011;32(6):751–9.
24. Enriquez-Sarano M, Suri RM, Clavel MA, Mantovani F, Michelena HI, Pislaru S, et al. Is there an outcome penalty linked to guideline-based indications for valvular surgery? Early and long-term analysis of patients with organic mitral regurgitation. J Thorac Cardiovasc Surg. 2015;150(1):50–8.
25. Suri RM, Vanoverschelde JL, Grigioni F, Schaff HV, Tribouilloy C, Avierinos JF, et al. Association between early surgical intervention vs watchful waiting and outcomes for mitral regurgitation due to flail mitral valve leaflets. JAMA. 2013;310(6):609–16.
26. Tribouilloy C, Rusinaru D, Grigioni F, Michelena HI, Vanoverschelde JL, Avierinos JF, et al. Long-term mortality associated with left ventricular dysfunction in mitral regurgitation due to flail leaflets: a multicenter analysis. Circ Cardiovasc Imaging. 2014;7(2):363–70.
27. Dziadzko V, Clavel MA, Dziadzko M, Medina-Inojosa JR, Michelena H, Maalouf J, et al. Outcome and undertreatment of mitral regurgitation: a community cohort study. Lancet. 2018;391(10124):960–9.
28. Iung B, Delgado V, Lazure P, Murray S, Sirnes PA, Rosenhek R, et al. Educational needs and application of guidelines in the management of patients with mitral regurgitation. A European mixed-methods study. Eur Heart J. 2018;39(15):1295–303.
29. Nashef SA, Roques F, Michel P, Gauducheau E, Lemeshow S, Salamon R. European system for cardiac operative risk evaluation (EuroSCORE). Eur J Cardiothorac Surg. 1999;16(1):9–13.
30. Nashef SA, Roques F, Sharples LD, Nilsson J, Smith C, Goldstone AR, et al. EuroSCORE II. Eur J Cardiothorac Surg. 2012;41(4):734–44.
31. O'Brien SM, Shahian DM, Filardo G, Ferraris VA, Haan CK, Rich JB, et al. The Society of Thoracic Surgeons 2008 cardiac surgery risk models: part 2—isolated valve surgery. Ann Thorac Surg. 2009;88(1 Suppl):S23–42.
32. Roques F, Nashef SA, Michel P, Gauducheau E, de Vincentiis C, Baudet E, et al. Risk factors and outcome in European cardiac surgery: analysis of the EuroSCORE multinational database of 19030 patients. Eur J Cardiothorac Surg. 1999;15(6):816–22.
33. Mirabel M, Iung B, Baron G, Messika-Zeitoun D, Detaint D, Vanoverschelde JL, et al. What are the characteristics of patients with severe, symptomatic, mitral regurgitation who are denied surgery? Eur Heart J. 2007;28(11):1358–65.
34. Lancellotti P, Rosenhek R, Pibarot P, Iung B, Otto CM, Tornos P, et al. ESC working group on valvular heart disease position paper—heart valve clinics: organization, structure, and experiences. Eur Heart J. 2013;34(21):1597–606.

Do We Need Heart Teams for Complex Cardiac Arrhythmias? A Cardiologist's Perspective

5

Mark Ainslie, Jennifer L. Reed, Krystina B. Lewis, and David Hugh Birnie

Introduction

In many academic cardiovascular centers, there has been a long-standing tradition of collaboration in the management of patients with complex arrhythmias. More recently, there have been initiatives at our institution and others to extend this further, i.e., create a formal "heart team" approach. Europe is leading the way in the heart team concept for management of arrhythmias; in a recent European survey of major cardiac centers, more than 95% of respondents felt an arrhythmia team was helpful, particularly in the management of complex arrhythmias, and arrhythmia teams had been established in 21 European centers [1]. Some of the complex arrhythmia heart team members at our institution are shown in Table 5.1. The ultimate goal is to provide high-quality, evidence-based, timely, cost-effective, personalized care to patients with complex arrhythmias.

M. Ainslie
Lancashire Cardiac Centre, Department of Cardiac Electrophysiology, Blackpool, UK

J. L. Reed
University of Ottawa Heart Institute, Department of Exercise Physiology and Cardiovascular Health Lab, Division of Cardiac Prevention and Rehabilitation, Ottawa, ON, Canada

K. B. Lewis
University of Ottawa School of Nursing, Ottawa, ON, Canada

D. H. Birnie (✉)
Division of Cardiology, University of Ottawa Heart Institute, Ottawa, ON, Canada
e-mail: dbirnie@ottawaheart.ca

© Springer Nature Switzerland AG 2019
T. Mesana (ed.), *Heart Teams for Treatment of Cardiovascular Disease*,
https://doi.org/10.1007/978-3-030-19124-5_5

47

Table 5.1 Complex arrhythmia heart team members

Complex arrhythmia	Heart team function	Heart team members
Atrial fibrillation (AF)	AF clinic	Nurses, interventional electrophysiologists, and cardiologists with interest in AF
	Decision-making about AF ablation	Interventional electrophysiologists, cardiac surgeons
	Prevention and management of postcardiac surgery AF	Cardiac surgeons, intensivists, electrophysiologists
	Decision-making about left atrial appendage (LAA) occlusion	Electrophysiologists Interventional cardiologists Imaging physicians
	Cardiac rehabilitation	Physiotherapists Exercise therapists
Ventricular arrhythmias	Ablation	Cardiac surgeons Interventional electrophysiologists
	VT management in left ventricular assist device (LVAD) patients	Cardiac surgeons Intensivists Interventional electrophysiologists Heart failure physicians
Inherited arrhythmia syndromes (IAS)	Inherited arrhythmia clinic	Arrhythmia specialists with training in IAS Nurses Medical geneticists Genetics counselors Psychologists/psychiatrists

Role of Heart Team for Management of Atrial Fibrillation

Epidemiology

Atrial fibrillation (AF) is the most commonly encountered rhythm disorder seen in clinical practice. Worldwide there are an estimated 21 million men and 12.6 million women with AF, and that number is set to increase [2, 3]. It is predicted that one-quarter of middle-aged adults in Europe and the United States will go on to develop AF [4]. The increasing prevalence of AF is in part due to an aging population with more predisposing comorbidities but also due to improved monitoring that detects asymptomatic AF [5]. AF is associated with both increased mortality and morbidity. There are a fivefold increased risk of stroke and a twofold increased risk of all-cause mortality due to sudden death, heart failure, and stroke in females and 1.5 times in males [4]. The economic burden of the disease is estimated to be between $6 and $26 billion US annually, made up of treatment costs and AF-related complications, in particular stroke [6].

Heart Team Approach to AF Clinic

AF is seen in many internal medicine and cardiology settings. There is growing evidence that the management of AF requires an integrated approach where modifiable

Table 5.2 European Society of Cardiology and National Institute of Clinical Effectiveness (UK) guidance on complex arrhythmia care

ESC—identified priority areas in heart team arrhythmia management	NICE (UK)—guidance on personalized package of care for AF patients
1. Patient involvement—patients are informed and involved in their care	1. Stroke awareness and measures to prevent stroke
2. Multidisciplinary team	2. Rate control/rhythm control
3. Use of modern technology Monitoring Delivery of information Decision support aids	3. Who to contact for advice if needed and psychological support if needed
4. Access to all treatments	Up-to-date and comprehensive education of patients and support networks (e.g., cardiovascular charities)

risk factors can be addressed and active therapy (medications and/or ablation) can be started. It has been shown that AF is often inadequately managed due to nonadherence to guidelines, with underuse of anticoagulation and inconsistent approach to risk factor reduction [4]. It has also been shown that an integrated and structured approach to AF care facilitates more consistent adherence to guidelines, with the potential to improve outcomes [7, 8]. Recent guidelines from the European Society of Cardiology (ESC) highlight four key areas for integrated AF management [4], while the National Institute of Clinical Effectiveness (NICE) in the United Kingdom published guidance in 2014 recommending a personalized package of care for AF patients [9]. A summary of their guidance is shown in Table 5.2.

In cardiovascular disease in general, specialist clinics have been shown to reduce all-cause mortality, rate of major cardiac events, and adherence to medication [10]. In heart failure, the role of the multidisciplinary team approach to outpatient clinics is very well established [11, 12]. Telemonitoring with the use of specialized nurses is seen to reduce mortality compared to standard clinic follow-up [13].

There are recent data to suggest that a similar heart team approach to AF outpatient care can lead to substantial patient benefits. Hendricks et al. [14] from the Netherlands randomly assigned 712 patients to AF clinic care versus usual care. AF clinic care consisted of a nurse-led clinic, supported by a dedicated software system based on ESC guidelines, and supervised by a cardiologist. In the clinic, the specialist nurse obtained a detailed patient history and educated the patient about the condition and reviewed test results. The patients were fully educated about anticoagulation and when to present to hospital. The software developed an individual patient profile based on the symptoms, risk factors, and type of AF. The software also proposed management options, which the nurse then discussed with the patient. A supervising cardiologist then approved the final treatment plan. The initial visit lasted 30 minutes, and this was followed up with visits at 3, 6, and 12 months and then every 6 months. Additional clinic visits and telephone consults were also used. The usual care cohort had a 20-minute consultation with a cardiologist and 10 minutes for follow-up visits [14]. A number of positive outcomes were noted. The primary outcome was a composite of cardiovascular hospitalization and death, and it occurred in 14.3% of patients in the AF clinic group compared with 20.8% in the control group. This equates to a 35% relative risk

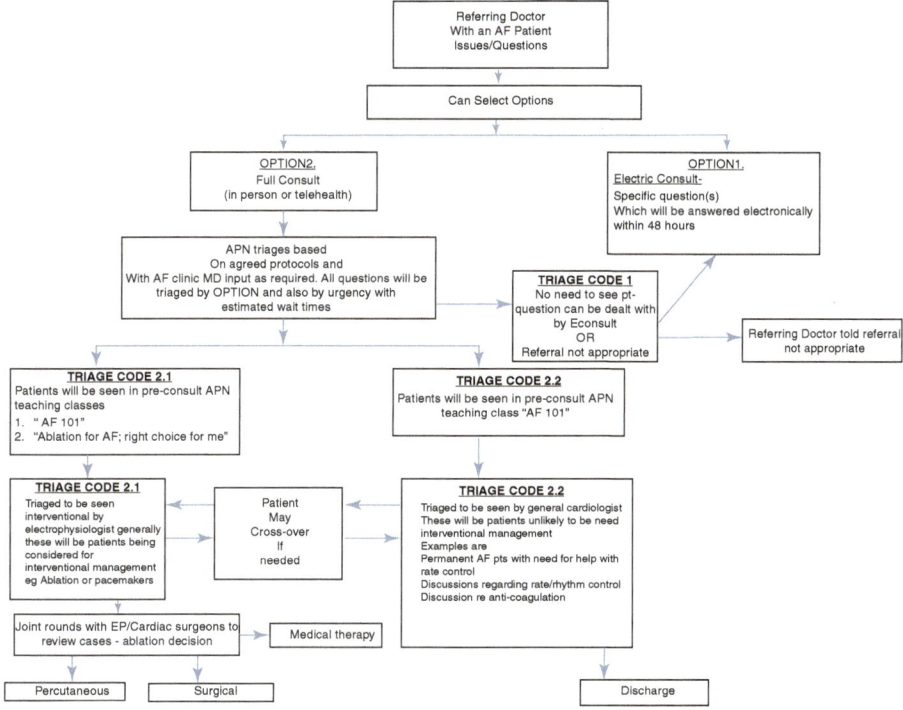

Fig. 5.1 Heart team AF clinic: University of Ottawa Heart Institute model

reduction [14]. Further studies by the same group have demonstrated increased patient knowledge regarding AF [15]. And a cost analysis of this patient cohort found the nurse-led care team saved 1109 Euros per patient compared to usual care [16].

In Australia, a home-based, disease-specific management for elderly chronic AF patients provided by specialist cardiac nurses, as part of a multidisciplinary team approach, had a positive impact in reducing the cardiovascular hospital stay (Fig. 5.1) [17].

Exercise Therapy, Risk Factor Modification, and Cardiac Rehabilitation for Patients with AF

AF-related symptoms may be disabling and highly variable. They include palpitations, fatigue, exercise intolerance, labored breathing, dizziness, diaphoresis, chest discomfort, sleep disturbances, anxiety, and depression, leading to decreases in quality of life (QoL) [18–24]. Growing research has examined the role of lifestyle interventions (i.e., exercise-based programs, aggressive risk factor modification, and cardiac rehabilitation [CR]) in managing the physical and mental health of patients with AF.

Exercise-Based Programs

Several reviews have examined the impact of exercise-based interventions in patients with AF [25–28]. Reed et al. in a systematic review ($N = 8$ studies) showed that chronic exercise training of continuous low, moderate, and vigorous intensity in patients with permanent AF significantly improved ventricular rate control, functional capacity, muscular strength and power, activities of daily living, and QoL [25]. Giacomantonio et al. in a systematic review demonstrated that moderate-intensity physical activity improved exercise capacity, activities of daily living, and QoL in patients with AF ($N = 6$ studies) [26]. Risom et al. in a Cochrane review ($N = 6$ randomized controlled trials) reported that exercise-based rehabilitation (i.e., comprising aerobic, resistance or interval training, Qi-gong, or inspiratory muscle training) has a clinically relevant impact on QoL, and may increase exercise capacity in patients with AF [27]. Most recently, Skielboe et al. reported that 12-week high-intensity and low-intensity interventions comprising twice-weekly exercise sessions similarly reduced AF burden in patients with PAF or permanent AF [29].

Risk Factor Modification

Emerging evidence suggests that risk factor modification improves clinical outcomes in patients with symptomatic paroxysmal AF (PAF) or persistent AF (perAF). In a landmark trial, Abed et al. [30] showed that weight reduction with intensive cardiometabolic risk factor (i.e., hypertension, hyperlipidemia, glucose intolerance, sleep apnea, and alcohol and tobacco use) management reduced AF symptom burden and severity and improved cardiac structure. In the ARREST-AF study, weight reduction with aggressive risk factor modification improved the long-term success of catheter ablation [31]. In the subsequent CARDIO-FIT trial, increased cardiorespiratory fitness was found to be synergistic with weight loss as part of the management strategy for rhythm control in overweight and obese patients with AF [32]. Lastly, in the LEGACY study, long-term sustained weight loss was associated with significant reduction of AF burden and maintenance of sinus rhythm in overweight and obese patients with AF; body mass fluctuations of >5% were associated with a greater likelihood of recurrent AF [33].

Cardiac Rehabilitation

Several investigators have examined the impact of cardiac rehabilitation (CR) on the physical health of patients with AF [34–36]. In patients with perAF and concomitant heart failure, Rienstra et al. showed that CR and targeted therapy of underlying conditions (i.e., mineralocorticoid receptor antagonists, statins, and angiotensin-converting enzyme inhibitors and angiotensin receptor blockers) for 1 year produced a modest but more successful modification in body mass index (0.12% vs. 1.37%) and significantly greater improvements in systolic (−3.28% vs. +2.05%)

and diastolic (−8.95% vs. −2.31%) blood pressure, total cholesterol (−13.21% vs. +1.65%), and low-density lipoprotein (−18.37% vs. +0.40%) when compared to conventional therapy [34]. Targeted therapy also significantly improved the maintenance of sinus rhythm (75% vs. 63%, OR = 1.765) when compared to conventional therapy, despite no difference in the rates of electrical cardioversion or use of anti-arrhythmic drugs between groups [34]. The risk of hospitalization and all-cause mortality was, however, similar between patients participating in targeted and conventional therapy [34].

In patients with PAF or perAF treated with catheter ablation, Risom et al. reported significantly greater improvements in VO$_2$ peak at 4 months of a 6-month CR program comprising thrice-weekly exercise training for 3 months and four psychoeducational sessions when compared to usual care (CR: 22.1–24.3 mL/kg/min vs. usual care: 22.1–20.7 mL/kg/min) [35]. Patients with an I–II European Heart Rhythm Association (EHRA) score were more likely to increase their VO$_2$ peak following CR when compared to those with an III–IV EHRA score (greater scores indicate more severe symptoms) [36]. Significantly greater improvements in functional capacity, as measured by 6-minute walk test distance, in CR vs. usual care at 4 months (CR: 548–592 m vs. usual care: 559–576 m) were also observed [35]. Sex-based analyses demonstrated that these differences were significant only among women [36].

Fewer investigators have examined the impact of CR on the mental health of patients with AF [35, 36]. In patients with PAF or perAF treated with catheter ablation, Risom et al. reported significantly greater improvements in self-reported general health (+6.84 vs. −1.61 points), but not in the Physical Component Summary or the Mental Component Summary scores, as measured by the Medical Outcomes study Short-From 36, following a 6-month CR program when compared to usual care [35]. Overall, anxiety and depression severity did not improve following 6 months of CR or usual care [35]. Wagner et al. performed secondary sex-based analyses and found significant improvements in anxiety severity in men, and global and treatment concern scores, as measured by the AF Quality-of-Life questionnaire, in women at 4 months of the 6-month CR program [36].

Future Directions

Research examining the impact of lifestyle interventions in patients with AF is growing. Exercise-based programs and CR may play an increasing role in managing the physical and mental health challenges in patients with AF. However, the findings to date are based on few studies with small sample sizes, varying AF populations, and moderate- to very low-quality evidence. Larger, adequately powered random controlled trials (RCTs) are needed to confirm these findings. Future trials should include (1) outcomes that matter most to patients (i.e., mortality, adverse events, and health-related QoL); (2) long-term outcomes to assess if short-term gains are maintained; (3) sex- and gender-based analyses; and (4) greater rigor in the reporting of

intervention details using reporting guidelines and checklists [37]. Given the initial successes with aggressive risk factor modification, future trials that include CR should not only evaluate the impact of exercise training, but also risk factor modification and psychosocial interventions, given the frequently reported poor mental health and QoL of patients with AF [18, 20–24].

Treatment Options for Patients with AF

Rate or Rhythm Control for AF

The decision to adopt a rhythm control or rate control strategy depends on a number of factors. There is no doubt that restoration of sinus rhythm improves cardiac hemodynamics and can improve symptoms of heart failure, improve quality of life, and may reverse some of the deleterious effects of atrial remodeling. However, there have been a number of randomized trials that have shown maintaining a rhythm control approach does not improve survival or reduce the risk of stroke in AF [38, 39]. A rate control approach aims to prevent rapid ventricular rate in AF. The drugs that can be used for this include beta-blockers, calcium channel blockers, digoxin, and, occasionally, amiodarone.

A rhythm control approach may involve an electrical cardioversion, antiarrhythmic drugs, and/or catheter ablation. The choice of approach is guided by patient symptom burden, chance of success of a rhythm control approach, and patient preferences. Indeed, a decision to initiate a rhythm control strategy depends on a careful balance between symptom burden, adverse drug effects, and patient choice.

Percutaneous Ablation: Techniques and Results

Percutaneous catheter ablation has developed over the last two decades from a specialized, experimental procedure into the most common invasive approach to manage AF. Percutaneous ablation is aimed at eliminating the potential triggers and/or modifying the arrhythmogenic substrate [40]. Almost 20 years ago, the basis for the catheter ablation was established with the observation that focal ectopic beats seen to be originating from the four pulmonary veins (PVs) were capable of triggering AF. Now the most commonly employed technique in modern ablation is the electrical isolation of the PVs by a circumferential ablation around the ostia of the four PVs (Fig. 5.2).

Alternative energy modalities are cryoenergy and laser, both applied by balloon-tipped catheters. To confirm pulmonary vein isolation, mapping catheters are placed within the veins to detect any residual electrical signals. Most procedures are performed using a combination of fluoroscopy, 3D electroanatomical mapping systems, and intracardiac ultrasound. Magnetic resonance imaging (MRI) and computed tomography (CT) images can also be integrated into modern systems. While

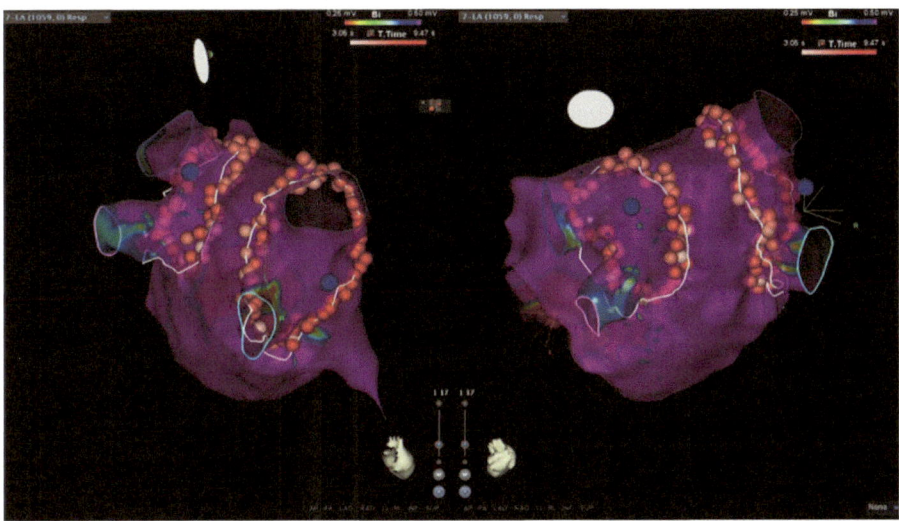

Fig. 5.2 3D generated map of the left atria and four pulmonary veins demonstrating ablations lesions for a wide antral circumferential ablation (WACA)

catheter ablation is a challenging and complex procedure, with a potential for life-threatening complications, through highly trained teams, it can be performed effectively and safely.

The most widely practiced ablation technique consists of a series of point-to-point radiofrequency (RF) lesions that encircle each set of veins. The most common method of delivering energy for ablative lesions is using a transvenous-irrigated RF catheter inserted via the femoral vein [41].

There are multiple definitions of procedural success. To the patient, a major reduction in symptoms due to AF is usually considered a success. In the clinical trial world, the usual "gold standard" definition of success is being free of clinical AF (<30 seconds) off antiarrhythmic medications. Using this latter definition two large meta-analyses of AF showed a single-procedure success of percutaneous ablation was 52% and a multiple-procedure success rate 71%, both off antiarrhythmic medications [42]. Although the distinction between paroxysmal AF (PAF) and persistent AF (perAF) was made, they were not analyzed separately. In a later meta-analysis, the procedural success was grouped by AF type. For PAF, single-procedure success was 68.6% (95% CI 58.9–77.0%) at 1 year; 61.1% (95% CI 49.8–71.2%) at 3 years; and 62.3% (95% CI 39.8–80.5%) at 5 years. For perAF, single-procedure success was 50.8% (95% CI 34.3–67.2%) at 1 year and 41.6% (95% CI 24.7–60.8%) at 3 years [43].

Stand-Alone Surgical AF Ablation: Techniques and Results

Many techniques have evolved over the years to be performed as a sole treatment for AF in the absence of other cardiac surgery. Williams et al. developed the first

approach in 1980, where a left-sided arteriotomy incision was described [44]. In 1985, Guiraudon et al. described the "corridor" technique whereby the part of the atrial septum containing the sinoatrial (SA) and atrioventricular (AV) node is isolated so that the SA node would be able to initiate ventricular contraction. This technique was generally not successful in maintaining sinus rhythm and, in fact, the excluded atrial areas outside the corridor often fibrillated, and risk of thromboembolism is high.

The major pioneer in surgical AF ablation was James Cox, with the initial development of the Cox-Maze procedure in 1991 [45]. The concept was based around the fact that splitting of the atrial tissue into smaller segments would prevent multiple re-entry wavelets to be maintained, and that the segments should be linked together to still allow depolarization of sufficient atrial myocardium. The procedure involved biatrial excisions with complete isolation of the each vein, an incision starting in the RA and extending across the fossa ovalis, a mitral isthmus incision, and cryoablation in the coronary sinus [45]. The Maze procedure has continued to evolve through versions II–IV. The success rates have been reported to range between 70% and 90%, with an operative mortality between 2% and 3% [46, 47]. Due to its complexity, requirement for aortic cross-clamp and cardiopulmonary bypass, it has not been widely adopted. A simplified version IV replaced the incisions with linear ablation lines using either RF, cryrothermy, or microwave energy. This can be performed through a small right thoracotomy, but cardiopulmonary bypass is still required [48].

Minimally invasive surgical techniques have been developed, and pulmonary vein isolation (PVI) and appendage removal are both possible with these approaches. A minimally invasive approach on a beating heart by Wolf et al.—where bilateral thoroscopy was used to perform a PVI and remove the left atrial appendage (LAA)—reported 91% of patients in sinus rhythm at 3 months [49]. In addition to the PVI, both ganglionic ablation and additional linear lines can be performed. With just the addition of ganglionic ablation, the 1-year freedom from AF has been reported to be between 75% and 87%, but these are nonrandomized trials [48]. One randomized trial by Boersma et al. compared minimally invasive ablation to percutaneous ablation in those who had failed previous RF ablation. The surgical procedure had a higher success rate, but at the cost of a substantially greater adverse event rate (23%) [50].

Concomitant Surgical AF Ablation: Techniques and Results

Up to 50% of patients undergoing heart surgery, in particular mitral valve surgery, have a history of AF [51]. A meta-analysis of nine RCTs including 472 patients, of whom 249 underwent a Maze procedure, found that performing a Maze at the time of concomitant surgery was associated with an increase in freedom from AF at 12 months. After excluding three studies that did not report freedom from AF within 12 months and a study that included PAF and perAF patients, 70.3% of patients in the MAZE group were free from AF at 12 months, and in the control group 31% were free of AF. Many of the studies included patients still on

antiarrhythmics, with only two giving results off medications. These two studies showed a much lower success rate, with 33% of patients in MAZE group free from AF at 12 months and 22% in the control group. With regard to safety, the overall rate of major complications was comparable, 24.4% in treatment group versus 24.9% control. Likewise, operative mortality was similar, with 4% in the treatment and 3.3% in the control [52].

Hybrid AF Ablation: Techniques, Results, and Future Directions

Great progress has been made in the last 25 years in both surgical and catheter-based ablation techniques. While the success rates for PAF have improved greatly [53], the success rates for patients with long-standing perAF remain low [54]. Surgical and percutaneous approaches have their own unique strengths, and there are many potential advantages of a hybrid ablation approach to patients with long-standing persistent AF (Table 5.3) and some teams have worked together to develop a hybrid AF ablation approach. This requires a strong collaborative approach between cardiac surgeons, electrophysiologists, and their respective teams.

Hybrid AF ablation consists of a surgical catheter ablation, usually applied via a minimally invasive thoracoscopically based approach, followed by a percutaneous ablation [55]. The percutaneous endocardial approach allows more complex mapping of the left atrium (LA) by the electrophysiologist, identifying any gaps in the ablation lesion sets and access to areas such as the mitral isthmus and cavotricuspid isthmus, which are technically difficult to access epicardially. Feedback to the surgeon with regard to the lesion sets likely will improve surgical results in this expanding field [55].

There have been a number of variations to the technique of the hybrid AF ablation, including surgical access, energy source, the timing of the two components, the ablation lesion set, and whether the left atrial appendage is excised or not. All,

Table 5.3 Relative advantages of surgical and catheter-based AF ablation strategies

Surgical	Catheter component
LA appendage exclusion	Endocardial mapping to ensure vein isolation and block across linear lines
Direct visualization of antrum of pulmonary veins	Identify gaps in lesion sets that require further epicardial ablation
Avoiding esophagus, phrenic nerve	Provide endocardial ablation to sites inaccessible from the epicardium, e.g., coronary sinus, cavotricuspid isthmus
Access to epicardial structures such as ganglionated plexi and ligament of Marshall	Mapping of rotors and CAFES
	Identification of endocardial and epicardial scar

however, do follow the main principle that there is an epicardial PVI with LA linear lines followed by an endocardial assessment of conduction block with additional ablations as required. A thoracoscopic approach uses bipolar RF and accesses the left atrium through the left and right pleura. A pericardioscopic approach uses monopolar RF and access to the LA is through the diaphragm or subxiphoid access [55]. The current evidence to support the safety and feasibility of this approach comes from mainly single-center observational studies. A meta-analysis of 16 suitable hybrid ablation studies including 785 patients found that 73% of all patients were in sinus rhythm off antiarrhythmics at the end of the follow-up period [56]. The overall short-term rate of significant complications was found to be 4%, which is lower than previously reported analyses. One important point was that there were three reported fatal atrial-esophageal cases.

A hybrid approach does have some limitations and challenges. If performed as a staged procedure, the endocardial mapping cannot guide further epicardial ablation. Since both epicardial and endocardial access is being obtained, the patient is exposed to the risks of both procedures and their associated morbidities. The logistics involved in coordinating the surgical and electrophysiology teams is not easy, as is the management of anticoagulation with healing surgical incisions. Finally, a staged approach also confers extra costs and recovery for the patient for two procedures. This will hopefully be offset by a reduction in the need for subsequent re-do procedures. Hybrid ablation is still in the early phases, and at present, there is no standard approach to it. There are two prospective, multicenter, industry-sponsored clinical trials of hybrid ablation underway: CONVERGE (NCT01984346) and DEEP (NCT01246466). The results of these will help guide the future direction of this new technique.

Current Guidelines to Direct Choice of Ablation Approach

The 2017 HRS guidelines give clear recommendations for both the use of percutaneous and surgical approaches for AF ablation [6]. These are summarized in Table 5.4.

Left Atrial Appendage Occlusion

Evidence suggests that the left atrial appendage (LAA) is implicated as the source of thrombus in more than 90% of strokes in AF [57]. The exclusion of the LAA would therefore be an attractive option in those patients unable or unwilling to take anticoagulation. The appendage was often excluded as part of the Cox-Maze procedure surgically, but more recently, there has been significant innovation in nonsurgical methods for occlusion of the LAA. There is an unmet clinical need for this alternative option for stroke prevention. Warfarin has a narrow therapeutic window, requires monitoring, and has many drug and food interactions. The novel oral anticoagulants (NOACs) have been shown to be noninferior in terms of stroke, but they

are more expensive and have high discontinuation rates ranging between 17% and 25% at 2 years, often due to bleeding complications [58–60].

The first LAA closure device was the PLAATO system in 2001. There are multiple devices currently available, and these can be classed as either endocardial plugs to occlude the LAA at the ostium, or epicardial ligation devices to exclude the LAA. The most widely studied and used device in clinical practice is the Watchman, which has been evaluated in two RCTs. The PROTECT-AF study demonstrated noninferiority versus warfarin for the primary efficacy rate and confirmed long-term safety. However, there was an increase in acute complications, including pericardial effusion and ischemic strokes (10.2% vs. 6.8%) [61]. The PREVAIL

Table 5.4 The 2017 HRS guidelines for the use of percutaneous and surgical approaches for AF ablation

Indications for percutaneous catheter ablation		Class of indication
Symptomatic AF refractory or intolerant to at least class I or III antiarrhythmic medication	Paroxysmal: catheter ablation is recommended	I
	Persistent: catheter ablation is reasonable	IIa
	Long-standing persistent: catheter ablation may be considered	IIb
Symptomatic AF prior to initiation of antiarrhythmic therapy with a class I or III antiarrhythmic medication	Paroxysmal: Catheter ablation is reasonable	IIa
	Persistent: Catheter ablation is reasonable	IIa
	Long-standing persistent: Catheter ablation may be considered	IIb
Indications for surgical ablation of AF		
Indications for concomitant open surgical ablation of AF (MVR)		
Symptomatic AF refractory or intolerant to at least one class I or III antiarrhythmic medication	Paroxysmal: Surgical ablation is recommended	I
	Persistent: Surgical ablation is recommended	I
	Long-standing persistent: Surgical ablation is recommended	I
Symptomatic AF prior to initiation of antiarrhythmic therapy with a class I or III antiarrhythmic medication	Paroxysmal: Surgical ablation is recommended	I
	Persistent: Surgical ablation is recommended	I
	Long-standing persistent: Surgical ablation is recommended	I
Indications for concomitant closed surgical ablation of AF (CABG/AVR)		
Symptomatic AF refractory or intolerant to at least one class I or III antiarrhythmic medication	Paroxysmal: Surgical ablation is recommended	I
	Persistent: Surgical ablation is recommended	I
	Long-standing persistent: Surgical ablation is recommended	I
Symptomatic AF prior to initiation of antiarrhythmic medication	Paroxysmal: Surgical ablation is reasonable	IIa
	Persistent: Surgical ablation is reasonable	IIa
	Long-standing persistent: Surgical ablation is reasonable	IIa

Table 5.4 (continued)

Indications for percutaneous catheter ablation		Class of indication
Indications for stand-alone and hybrid surgical ablation of AF		
Symptomatic AF refractory or intolerant to at least one class I or III antiarrhythmic medication	Paroxysmal: Stand-alone surgical ablation can be considered for patients who have previously failed catheter ablation and also for those who are intolerant or refractory to antiarrhythmic drug therapy and prefer a surgical approach, after review of the relative safety and efficacy of catheter ablation versus a stand-alone surgical approach	IIb
	Persistent: Stand-alone surgical ablation is reasonable for patients who have previously failed catheter ablation and also for those patients who prefer a surgical approach after review of the relative safety and efficacy of catheter ablation versus a stand-alone surgical approach	IIa
	Long-standing persistent: Stand-alone surgical ablation is reasonable for patients who have previously failed catheter ablation and also for those patients who prefer a surgical approach after review of the relative safety and efficacy of catheter ablation versus a stand-alone surgical approach	IIa
	It might be reasonable to apply the indications for stand-alone surgical ablation described above to patients being considered for hybrid surgical AF ablation	IIb

study further reinforced efficacy data, and with more training, acute complications were shown to be reduced [62]. The EVOLUTION registry with over 1000 patients has shown a procedural success of 98.5%, with a 30-day mortality of 0.7%. The Amplatzer device is relatively simple to use and its use is widespread in closing septal defects. There have been no randomized trials for its use in LAA occlusion, but the largest retrospective study included 1047 patients from Europe and Canada and showed a 97.3% procedure success rate with a 1-year mortality of 4.2%, with an approximately 60% risk reduction in both systemic thromboembolism and major bleeding [63].

Currently due to limited data from clinical trials, guideline recommendations for LAA occlusion devices are limited. Neither Canadian nor US guidelines specify indications for their use. The 2016 ESC guidelines give a class IIb indication for percutaneous LAA closure in patients who are at high risk of stroke and who have contraindications to long-term anticoagulation, i.e., specifically those with life-threatening bleed(s) with no reversible cause [4].

There has been a debate over whether this procedure should be done by structural interventionalists or by electrophysiologists. Both have unique skills sets,

with interventionalists more used to deployment of intracardiac devices and the electrophysiologist more used to transeptal puncture and left atrial anatomy. The American College of Cardiology (ACC) recommends that physicians performing these procedures have significant knowledge of AF and all its management, and have experience with left-sided cardiac procedures [64]. The LAA heart team ideally should include input from both disciplines along with imaging expertise prior to and during the procedure.

Role of the Heart Team for Management of Ventricular Arrhythmias

Ventricular tachycardia (VT) is classified into structurally normal versus structurally abnormal heart conditions and ischemic vs. nonischemic etiologies. The treatment of this has evolved over the years from the use of drugs, implantation of cardioverter defibrillators, and now percutaneous ablation. In the vast majority of cases, the mechanism of VT is due to re-entry around a region of scar [65]. The role of ablation is to target the critical areas of these circuits that can maintain the tachycardia [66].

Role of the Cardiac Surgeon in Assisting the Electrophysiologist in the Management of Ventricular Arrhythmias

Patients with life-threatening ventricular arrhythmias are perhaps the sickest patient cohorts encountered by the complex arrhythmia heart team. These patients usually require multidisciplinary expertise in their management. This heart team should include electrophysiologists, heart failure cardiologists, critical care intensivists, surgeons, and allied professionals. Some of the patients who require ablation are hemodynamically unstable, and they may require circulatory support during the ablation. This may take the form of cardiopulmonary bypass, extracorporeal membrane oxygenation (ECMO), percutaneous left ventricular devices (pLVADs), and surgical LVADs, all of which the surgical team can help provide. VT ablation has been shown to be successful with adjunctive support, and certainly allows the sickest of patients to be treated [67]. While many ablations can be performed endocardially, some VTs originate from the epicardium. While the epicardium can often be accessed percutaneously, this is not always the case, and the surgeon can help provide access to the pericardium [68].

Surgical VT Ablation

Historically, the only treatment option available to those patients with drug-refractory VT was to consider surgical options [69]. VT was an extremely common complication post myocardial infractions in the pre-thrombolysis and now pre-PCI

era, with full-thickness infarcts providing a large substrate for VT circuits. For those arrhythmias that were ischemic driven, the main treatment was revascularization with a coronary artery bypass. However, in cases with significant scarring, and in those where the ventricle is aneurysmal, VT was very likely to occur.

The concept of ablation to attempt a cure for ventricular arrhythmias evolved in the 1970s, and a variety of surgical procedures were developed. Since the VT was a direct result of scar tissue, surgical approaches focused on removal of the scar tissue. A number of techniques have been described in the literature, which include aneursymectomy, encircling endocardial ventriculotomy (EEV), partial EEV, endocardial resection (ER), cryoablation, or a combination of the above [70].

With the introduction of implantable cardioverter defibrillators (ICDs), more advanced medical therapies, and the development of catheter-based ablations, the need for surgical VT ablation as an isolated procedure declined greatly. Although now a rarely performed procedure, in the ischemic cohort of patients' interest in surgical ablation has increased in the nonischemic cardiomyopathy cohort. The scar distribution is very different from ischemic cardiomyopathy and highly variable. They are often perivalvular, intramural, and frequently epicardial. Failed catheter ablation in part is due to anatomical obstacles, intramural lesions may be too deep to penetrate, epicardial circuits may be protected by epicardial fat, or be too close to a coronary artery. The electrophysiology group at the University of Pennsylvania are world-renowned experts in the field of VT ablation. They are strong advocates of a team-based approach to VT, including the importance of surgical VT ablation in patients with a failed percutaneous approach [71, 72]. In their experience, preprocedural mapping can direct the surgeons' efforts, improving the effectiveness of the ablation. Twenty patients with NICM underwent surgical VT ablation with a VT-free survival at 1 year of 73% and a marked reduction in ICD therapies following the procedure [72]. These cases were all done with initial detailed mapping prior to the surgery as a separate procedure.

VT Management in Patients with Left Ventricular Assist Devices (LVADs)

LVADs are increasingly being used as a bridge to cardiac transplantation and, in some health systems, as a bridge to destination. Postoperative ventricular arrhythmias occur in up to 1/3 of patients within 30 days [73, 74]. Ventricular arrhythmias are often a bad prognostic sign if they occur within the first week, with a high mortality associated with it [75]. The VAs may be the result of persistent ischemia, acute off-loading using changes in repolarization, the ventricular remodeling process, fibrosis, the inotropic agents used, and the sewing ring used to secure the LVAD inflow cannula [76]. The management of VT in this situation greatly relies on a team-based approach and frequent discussions between electrophysiologists, heart failure/transplant cardiologists, critical care intensivists, and surgeons.

VT ablation has been shown to be effective and relatively safe in those with intractable VT, despite pharmacotherapy and treatment of all potential reversible

cause [76]. In one small case series, an open-chest hybrid epicardial ablation was performed on five patients for intractable VT post-LVAD with reasonable success [77]. In another case series of six patients, endocardial ablation was performed either transeptally or by a retrograde aortic approach. They found that VT was eliminated in four patients and the frequency of ICD shocks was markedly reduced in the remaining two patients [78]. In the majority of patients, medical management will be enough, but a coordinated team effort is clearly required.

Role of the Heart Team for Management of Inherited Arrhythmias

The diagnosis, risk stratification, and management of patients and their families affected by inherited primary arrhythmia syndromes can be very challenging. The inherited arrhythmia syndromes are usually classified as one of the following:

- Brugada syndrome
- Long and short QT syndrome
- Arrhythmogenic right ventricular cardiomyopathy
- Catecholaminergic polymorphic ventricular tachycardia
- Cardiac arrest of unknown cause

The rapid advancement in clinical genetics, combined with an overall low prevalence of these conditions, makes it difficult for a cardiologist or general electrophysiologist to gain enough exposure to gain and maintain expertise, and hence, specialist clinics have developed. Evidence suggests that a structured, multidisciplinary team-based approach improves the likelihood of making the correct diagnosis [79–81]. The ideal team should include a clinical cardiologist/electrophysiologist with a special interest in inherited arrhythmia alongside a medical geneticist and a genetics counselor, with intermittent access to specialized clinical psychologists, psychiatrists, and pharmacists [79].

Many patients will be survivors of sudden cardiac arrest, or family members of those with arrest and even death. This, combined with a potential diagnosis of an inherited disease, makes for a highly emotional time for those involved [82, 83]. Involvement of, or at least access to, psychologists and psychiatrists is therefore important. Ultimately, the aim of pooling expertise in one clinic is to improve the quality of delivered care, and improves patient outcomes at a lower overall cost [79]. Figure 5.3 shows recommended team-based approach to management of inherited arrhythmias (based on the 2013 HRS/EHRA/APHRS Expert Consensus Statement on the Diagnosis and Management of Patients with Inherited Primary Arrhythmia Syndromes) [79].

Physicians from our institution recently published their clinical experience with a team-based approach to inherited arrhythmias [84]. In over 700 patients, more than 1/3 of individuals had a diagnosis and received a long-term management plan. Compliance with medication was shown to be very high, and the event rate for

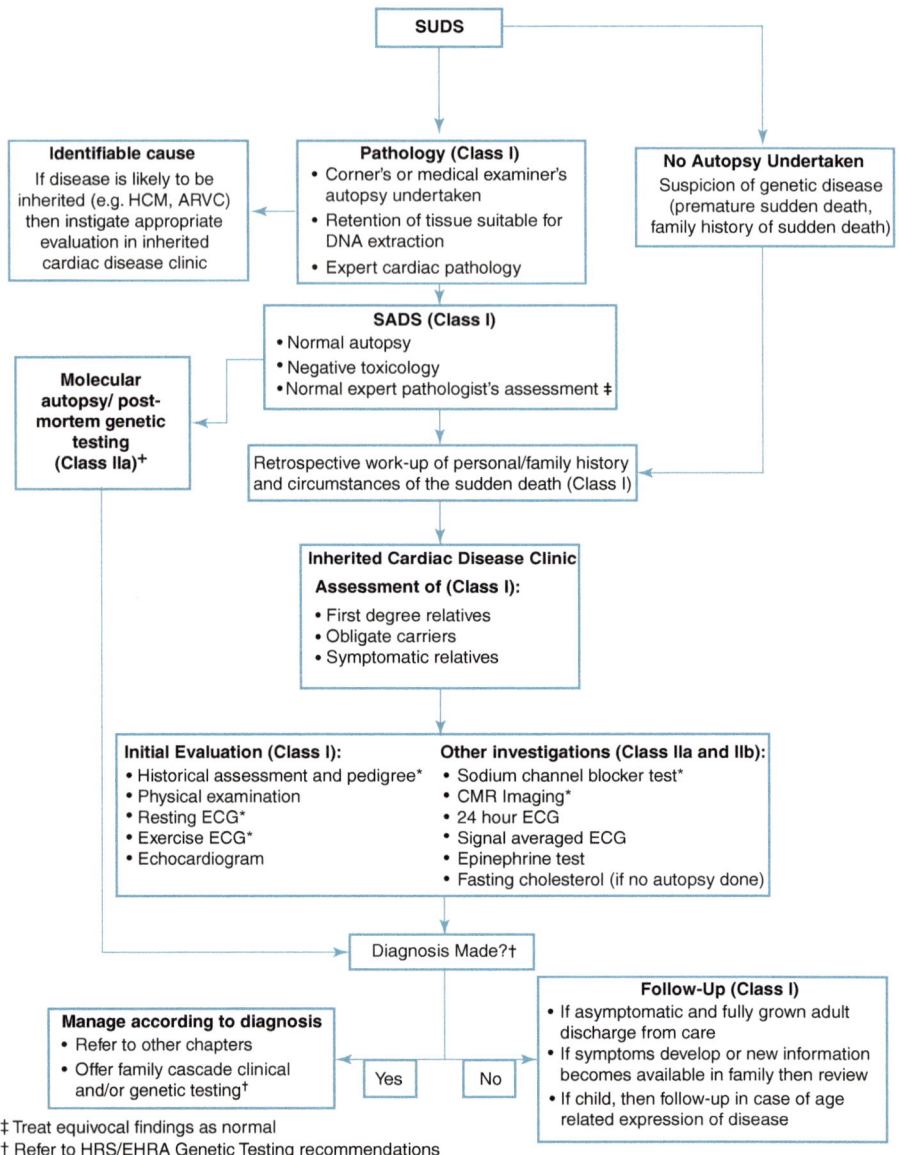

Fig. 5.3 HRS/EHRA/APHRS recommended team-based approach to management of inherited arrhythmias

serious arrhythmias was very low, with only one patient having sudden cardiac death (SCD) in the follow-up of over 5 years. Only 4% were deemed to require a primary prevention ICD, and with the very low event rate seen in the patients, we strongly support the idea that an expert clinic prevents the unnecessarily placement of devices and their potential associated morbidities [84].

The Patient as a Member of the Team: Shared Decision-Making for Patients with Complex Arrhythmias

The best treatment option for the individual patient with complex arrhythmias is not always clear, either because the evidence is insufficient, or there is a need to trade off benefits and risks. Active patient participation in health decisions is essential for patient-centered care. Shared decision-making (SDM), described as the pinnacle of patient-centered care [85], is a collaborative process that occurs between patients and clinicians whereby treatment decisions are made jointly by engaging in conversation about the best available evidence and patient preferences, deliberating about the pros and cons of each option, and arriving at a consensual decision [86, 87]. The goal for the practicing clinician is to increase the likelihood that the selected treatment is consistent with an informed patient's values and preferences. Increasingly, a SDM approach is recommended in clinical practice guidelines and expert consensus documents for the management of many patients with complex arrhythmias, including AF [88, 89], ventricular arrhythmias [90], and ICDs [91, 92].

Interventions to Facilitate Shared Decision-Making

Patient decision aids (PDAs), decision coaching, and question prompts sheets are evidence-based interventions, which can support a SDM process within or ahead of a clinical consultation [93–96]. PDAs are paper-based booklets, videos, or web-based materials designed to complement patient–clinician interactions [93]. At a minimum, PDAs explicitly state the decision to be made, provide information about the options (including status quo) and outcomes (e.g., benefits, harms) associated with each option, and help patients clarify their values and preferences [97]. Decision coaching is delivered by a trained healthcare provider and is a defined set of skills that is used to support patients in a nondirective manner to foster their active participation [96]. Question prompts are delivered before consultations and are designed to help patients identify their informational needs and list questions for their healthcare provider [95]. These three types of interventions enhance decision quality and decision-making processes, without harm (Table 5.5).

SDM for Patients with AF

A recent systematic review of formally evaluated PDAs for stroke prevention in AF identified seven studies. In six PDAs, treatment options included aspirin, warfarin, or no treatment. Only one PDA included a new oral anticoagulant, dabigatran, as a

Table 5.5 Effect of SDM interventions on decision quality and decision-making process outcomes

	PDA	Decision coaching	Question prompts
Decision quality outcomes			
Improve knowledge	√	√	
More accurate risk perception of outcomes	√		
Chosen option congruent with patients' values	√		
Decision-making process outcomes			
Less decisional conflict (uninformed, unclear values)	√		
Fewer remaining undecided	√		
Higher patient participation in decision-making	√	√	
Improved patient-clinician communication	√		√
Increased satisfaction		√	√

√ Statistically significant difference

treatment option alongside conventional therapies [98]. The PDAs were delivered in outpatient settings. None are publicly available. Newer digital PDAs are emerging as smartphone applications and some with electronic medical record compatibility; however, these have not been formally evaluated [99]. Current research is exploring the delivery of PDAs for anticoagulation for patients with new-onset AF presenting to the emergency department [99]. In practice in the United States, the Centers for Medicare and Medicaid Services provides reimbursement for percutaneous LAA closure devices for patients with nonvalvular AF on the condition that a formal SDM process occurred, evidenced by the documented use of a PDA on anticoagulation options with an independent noninterventional physician [100]. In June 2018, the Mayo Clinic and the University of Utah received research funding from the American Heart Association and the Patient-Centered Outcomes Research Institute to establish the Decision-making and Choices to Inform Dialogue and Empower AF Patients (DECIDE) Center, which will support the development or adaptation, evaluation, and implementation of decision support tools [101].

SDM for Patients with Cardiac Implantable Electronic Devices

SDM for cardiac implantable electronic devices (CIEDs) therapy has primarily focused on the series of decisions associated with ICD therapy, including the option to implant, replace, or deactivate therapies nearing patient end-of-life. Decisions regarding ICD therapy are considered iterative and ongoing, as patients' clinical status, life circumstances, and goals of care evolve. PDAs exist to accept or decline an ICD for primary prevention [102, 103]. A PDA with nurse-led decision coaching

for ICD pulse generator replacement was developed and pilot tested by an interprofessional team at the University of Ottawa Heart Institute [104]. And finally, with broad stakeholder involvement, Ontario's CorHealth developed a comprehensive ICD deactivation booklet for patients and families [105], and a companion guide for healthcare professionals, which recommends a SDM approach [106].

Future Directions

Until now, the development of SDM interventions has relied primarily on health research funding, an unreliable source for ongoing updates, and scaling-up and sustainability efforts [107]. Further, despite established benefits and effectiveness in research settings, their implementation in cardiac arrhythmia clinical practice is elusive [107]. Embedding decision support interventions in clinical practice can be facilitated by increased awareness for patients and healthcare professionals, access to high-quality SDM tools, formal clinician training, and organizational support [108, 109]. Also suggested is the development and validation of quality indicators supporting SDM practices, such as the documentation of patient preferences or PDA use for targeted decisions, yet further research is needed to measure the impact of such mandates on patient and system outcomes [110, 111]. As future studies contend with widening indications for cardiac arrhythmia therapies, interventions to support SDM at many decision points will become increasingly common and a vital component of the heart team-based approach to complex arrhythmias.

This heart team approach to complex arrhythmias at our institution has had some initial success. The team outcome metrics (currently active and proposed) are shown in Table 5.6.

Table 5.6 Heart team outcome metrics (currently active and proposed)

	Current metrics being collected	Metrics to be collected in future
AF	Wait times to be seen in AF clinic	Cost-effectiveness of AF clinic
	Wait times between AF clinic and ablation	Patient satisfaction and quality of life (generic and disease specific)
	Number of ER visits between referral and AF clinic and ablation	Before and after AF clinic
	Outcomes from AF ablation	Before and after ablation
	Complications from AF ablation	
	Mean number of AF ablations per patient	
	Heart team case conferences—outcomes	
	Rates of AF after cardiac surgery	
Ventricular arrhythmias	Wait times for ablation	
	Outcomes from ablation	
	Complications from ablation	
Inherited arrhythmias	Clinic wait times	Patient educational needs
	Patient long-term outcomes	Patient psychological outcomes

Conclusion

The complex arrhythmia heart team approach has already been shown to be cost-effective in a number of areas. Many European centers have adopted a multidisciplinary model, and the majority of physicians when surveyed felt this approach had a positive impact on patient care [1]. Examples of proven cost savings include dedicated AF clinic [16] and a coordinated approach to reduction of postcardiac surgery AF [112]. Additional potential savings could follow from:

(i)   Reduction of ER visits by fast-tracking of patients for ablation
(ii) Reduction of ER visits by rapid access AF clinics
(iii) Prevention of inappropriate ablation in patients with very little likelihood of success
(iv) Reduction of an appropriate testing and duplicate physician visits by rapid triage of patients to dedicated AF clinics

The hope is that the concept of the "complex arrhythmia heart team" will continue to evolve and grow at our institution and others. In our experience, the heart team approach has met with two main challenges. The first challenge has been broad physician engagement. The second issue has been to develop a sustainable economic model to support the team in the long term. Going forward, we hope to convince healthcare administrators and funders that savings achieved by the team should, at least in part, be directed to support the team. Meantime, we will continue to focus on our ultimate goal to provide high-quality, evidence-based, timely, cost-effective, personalized care to patients with complex arrhythmias.

References

1. Fumagalli S, Chen J, Dobreanu D, Madrid AH, Tilz R, Dagres N. The role of the arrhythmia team, an integrated, multidisciplinary approach to treatment of patients with cardiac arrhythmias: results of the European Heart Rhythm Association survey. Europace. 2016;18(4):623–7.
2. Chugh SS, Havmoeller R, Narayanan K, Singh D, Rienstra M, Benjamin EJ, et al. Worldwide epidemiology of atrial fibrillation: a Global Burden of Disease 2010 Study. Circulation. 2014;129(8):837–47.
3. Colilla S, Crow A, Petkun W, Singer DE, Simon T, Liu X. Estimates of current and future incidence and prevalence of atrial fibrillation in the U.S. adult population. Am J Cardiol. 2013;112(8):1142–7.
4. Kirchhof P, Benussi S, Kotecha D, Ahlsson A, Atar D, Casadei B, et al. 2016 ESC guidelines for the management of atrial fibrillation developed in collaboration with EACTS. Eur Heart J. 2016;37(38):2893–962.
5. Sanna T, Diener HC, Passman RS, Di Lazzaro V, Bernstein RA, Morillo CA, et al. Cryptogenic stroke and underlying atrial fibrillation. N Engl J Med. 2014;370(26):2478–86.
6. Calkins H, Hindricks G, Cappato R, Kim YH, Saad EB, Aguinaga L, et al. 2017 HRS/EHRA/ECAS/APHRS/SOLAECE expert consensus statement on catheter and surgical ablation of atrial fibrillation. Heart Rhythm. 2017;14(10):e275–444.
7. Berti D, Hendriks JM, Brandes A, Deaton C, Crijns HJ, Camm AJ, et al. A proposal for interdisciplinary, nurse-coordinated atrial fibrillation expert programmes as a way to structure daily practice. Eur Heart J. 2013;34(35):2725–30.

8. Nieuwlaat R, Olsson SB, Lip GY, Camm AJ, Breithardt G, Capucci A, et al. Guideline-adherent antithrombotic treatment is associated with improved outcomes compared with undertreatment in high-risk patients with atrial fibrillation. The Euro Heart Survey on Atrial Fibrillation. Am Heart J. 2007;153(6):1006–12.
9. Vizel' AA, Nasretdinova GR, Islamova LV, Vizel' EA. [Evaluation of the efficiency of various treatment regimens for patients with newly-detected sarcoidosis in the Republic of Tatarstan]. Probl Tuberk Bolezn Legk. 2006(4):19–23. [Article in Russian].
10. Al-Mallah MH, Farah I, Al-Madani W, Bdeir B, Al Habib S, Bigelow ML, et al. The impact of nurse-led clinics on the mortality and morbidity of patients with cardiovascular diseases: a systematic review and meta-analysis. J Cardiovasc Nurs. 2016;31(1):89–95.
11. Watanabe H, Chinushi M, Izumi D, Sato A, Okada S, Okamura K, et al. Decrease in amplitude of intracardiac ventricular electrogram and inappropriate therapy in patients with an implantable cardioverter defibrillator. Int Heart J. 2006;47(3):363–70.
12. Il'kovich MM, Perlei VE, Amosov VI, Lebedeva EV. [Early diagnosis of pulmonary hemodynamic disorders in patients with pulmonary sarcoidosis]. Probl Tuberk Bolezn Legk. 2006(4):45–50. [Article in Russian].
13. Hindricks G, Taborsky M, Glikson M, Heinrich U, Schumacher B, Katz A, et al. Implant-based multiparameter telemonitoring of patients with heart failure (IN-TIME): a randomised controlled trial. Lancet. 2014;384(9943):583–90.
14. Hendriks JM, de Wit R, Crijns HJ, Vrijhoef HJ, Prins MH, Pisters R, et al. Nurse-led care vs. usual care for patients with atrial fibrillation: results of a randomized trial of integrated chronic care vs. routine clinical care in ambulatory patients with atrial fibrillation. Eur Heart J. 2012;33(21):2692–9.
15. Hendriks JM, Vrijhoef HJ, Crijns HJ, Brunner-La Rocca HP. The effect of a nurse-led integrated chronic care approach on quality of life in patients with atrial fibrillation. Europace. 2014;16(4):491–9.
16. Hendriks J, Tomini F, van Asselt T, Crijns H, Vrijhoef H. Cost-effectiveness of a specialized atrial fibrillation clinic vs. usual care in patients with atrial fibrillation. Europace. 2013;15(8):1128–35.
17. Stewart S, Ball J, Horowitz JD, Marwick TH, Mahadevan G, Wong C, et al. Standard versus atrial fibrillation-specific management strategy (SAFETY) to reduce recurrent admission and prolong survival: pragmatic, multicentre, randomised controlled trial. Lancet. 2015;385(9970):775–84.
18. Gronefeld GC, Hohnloser SH. Quality of life in atrial fibrillation: an increasingly important issue. Eur Heart J Suppl. 2003;5:H25–33.
19. Healey JS, Parkash R, Pollak T, Tsang T, Dorian P, Committee CCSAFG. Canadian Cardiovascular Society atrial fibrillation guidelines 2010: etiology and initial investigations. Can J Cardiol. 2011;27(1):31–7.
20. Dabrowski R, Smolis-Bak E, Kowalik I, Kazimierska B, Wojcicka M, Szwed H. Quality of life and depression in patients with different patterns of atrial fibrillation. Kardiol Pol. 2010;68(10):1133–9.
21. Ariansen I, Dammen T, Abdelnoor M, Tveit A, Gjesdal K. Mental health and sleep in permanent atrial fibrillation patients from the general population. Clin Cardiol. 2011;34(5):327–31.
22. Thrall G, Lane D, Carroll D, Lip GY. Quality of life in patients with atrial fibrillation: a systematic review. Am J Med. 2006;119(5):448 e1–19.
23. Kang Y, Bahler R. Health-related quality of life in patients newly diagnosed with atrial fibrillation. Eur J Cardiovasc Nurs. 2004;3(1):71–6.
24. Dorian P, Jung W, Newman D, Paquette M, Wood K, Ayers GM, et al. The impairment of health-related quality of life in patients with intermittent atrial fibrillation: implications for the assessment of investigational therapy. J Am Coll Cardiol. 2000;36(4):1303–9.
25. Reed JL, Mark AE, Reid RD, Pipe AL. The effects of chronic exercise training in individuals with permanent atrial fibrillation: a systematic review. Can J Cardiol. 2013;29(12):1721–8.

26. Giacomantonio NB, Bredin SS, Foulds HJ, Warburton DE. A systematic review of the health benefits of exercise rehabilitation in persons living with atrial fibrillation. Can J Cardiol. 2013;29(4):483–91.
27. Risom SS, Zwisler AD, Johansen PP, Sibilitz KL, Lindschou J, Gluud C, et al. Exercise-based cardiac rehabilitation for adults with atrial fibrillation. Cochrane Database Syst Rev. 2017;2:CD011197.
28. Lowres N, Neubeck L, Freedman SB, Briffa T, Bauman A, Redfern J. Lifestyle risk reduction interventions in atrial fibrillation: a systematic review. Eur J Prev Cardiol. 2012;19(5):1091–100.
29. Skielboe AK, Bandholm TQ, Hakmann S, Mourier M, Kallemose T, Dixen U. Cardiovascular exercise and burden of arrhythmia in patients with atrial fibrillation—a randomized controlled trial. PLoS One. 2017;12(2):e0170060.
30. Abed HS, Wittert GA, Leong DP, Shirazi MG, Bahrami B, Middeldorp ME, et al. Effect of weight reduction and cardiometabolic risk factor management on symptom burden and severity in patients with atrial fibrillation: a randomized clinical trial. JAMA. 2013;310(19):2050–60.
31. Pathak RK, Middeldorp ME, Lau DH, Mehta AB, Mahajan R, Twomey D, et al. Aggressive risk factor reduction study for atrial fibrillation and implications for the outcome of ablation: the ARREST-AF cohort study. J Am Coll Cardiol. 2014;64(21):2222–31.
32. Pathak RK, Elliott A, Middeldorp ME, Meredith M, Mehta AB, Mahajan R, et al. Impact of CARDIOrespiratory FITness on arrhythmia recurrence in obese individuals with atrial fibrillation: the CARDIO-FIT study. J Am Coll Cardiol. 2015;66(9):985–96.
33. Pathak RK, Middeldorp ME, Meredith M, Mehta AB, Mahajan R, Wong CX, et al. Long-term effect of goal-directed weight management in an atrial fibrillation cohort: a long-term follow-up study (LEGACY). J Am Coll Cardiol. 2015;65(20):2159–69.
34. Rienstra M, Hobbelt AH, Alings M, Tijssen JGP, Smit MD, Brugemann J, et al. Targeted therapy of underlying conditions improves sinus rhythm maintenance in patients with persistent atrial fibrillation: results of the RACE 3 trial. Eur Heart J. 2018;01:01.
35. Risom SS, Zwisler AD, Rasmussen TB, Sibilitz KL, Madsen TLS, Svendsen JH, et al. Cardiac rehabilitation versus usual care for patients treated with catheter ablation for atrial fibrillation: results of the randomized CopenHeart. Am Heart J. 2016;181:120–9.
36. Wagner MK, Zwisler ADO, Risom SS, Svendsen JH, Christensen AV, Berg SK. Sex differences in health status and rehabilitation outcomes in patients with atrial fibrillation treated with ablation: results from the CopenHeartRFA trial. Eur J Cardiovasc Nurs. 2018;17(2):123–35.
37. Hoffmann TC, Glasziou PP, Boutron I, Milne R, Perera R, Moher D, et al. Better reporting of interventions: template for intervention description and replication (TIDieR) checklist and guide. BMJ. 2014;348:g1687.
38. Chatterjee S, Sardar P, Lichstein E, Mukherjee D, Aikat S. Pharmacologic rate versus rhythm-control strategies in atrial fibrillation: an updated comprehensive review and meta-analysis. Pacing Clin Electrophysiol. 2013;36(1):122–33.
39. Meyer T, Lauschke J, Ruppert V, Richter A, Pankuweit S, Maisch B. Isolated cardiac sarcoidosis associated with the expression of a splice variant coding for a truncated BTNL2 protein. Cardiology. 2008;109(2):117–21.
40. Allessie M, Ausma J, Schhotten U. Electrical, contractile and structural remodelling during atrial fibrillation. Cardiovasc Res. 2002;54(2):230–46.
41. Haegeli L. CardioPulse. Percutaneous radiofrequency catheter ablation of atrial fibrillation. Eur Heart J. 2012;33(21):2625–7.
42. Calkins H, Reynolds MR, Spector P, Sondhi M, Xu Y, Martin A, et al. Treatment of atrial fibrillation with antiarrhythmic drugs or radiofrequency ablation: two systematic literature reviews and meta-analyses. Circ Arrhythm Electrophysiol. 2009;2(4):349–61.
43. Ganesan AN, Shipp NJ, Brooks AG, Kuklik P, Lau DH, Lim HS, et al. Long-term outcomes of catheter ablation of atrial fibrillation: a systematic review and meta-analysis. J Am Heart Assoc. 2013;2(2):e004549.

44. Williams JM, Ungerleider RM, Lofland GK, Cox JL. Left atrial isolation: new technique for the treatment of supraventricular arrhythmias. J Thorac Cardiovasc Surg. 1980;80(3):373–80.
45. Cox JL. The surgical treatment of atrial fibrillation. IV. Surgical technique. J Thorac Cardiovasc Surg. 1991;101(4):584–92.
46. Damiano RJ Jr, Gaynor SL, Bailey M, Prasad S, Cox JL, Boineau JP, et al. The long-term outcome of patients with coronary disease and atrial fibrillation undergoing the Cox Maze procedure. J Thorac Cardiovasc Surg. 2003;126(6):2016–21.
47. Ballaux PK, Geuzebroek GS, van Hemel NM, Kelder JC, Dossche KM, Ernst JM, et al. Freedom from atrial arrhythmias after classic Maze III surgery: a 10-year experience. J Thorac Cardiovasc Surg. 2006;132(6):1433–40.
48. Fragakis N, Pantos I, Younis J, Hadjipavlou M, Katritsis DG. Surgical ablation for atrial fibrillation. Europace. 2012;14(11):1545–52.
49. Wolf RK, Schneeberger EW, Osterday R, Miller D, Merrill W, Flege JB Jr, et al. Video-assisted bilateral pulmonary vein isolation and left atrial appendage exclusion for atrial fibrillation. J Thorac Cardiovasc Surg. 2005;130(3):797–802.
50. Boersma LV, Castella M, van Boven W, Berruezo A, Yilmaz A, Nadal M, et al. Atrial fibrillation catheter ablation versus surgical ablation treatment (FAST): a 2-center randomized clinical trial. Circulation. 2012;125(1):23–30.
51. Cox JL. Intraoperative options for treating atrial fibrillation associated with mitral valve disease. J Thorac Cardiovasc Surg. 2001;122(2):212–5.
52. Kong MH, Lopes RD, Piccini JP, Hasselblad V, Bahnson TD, Al-Khatib SM. Surgical Maze procedure as a treatment for atrial fibrillation: a meta-analysis of randomized controlled trials. Cardiovasc Ther. 2010;28(5):311–26.
53. Kimura K, Tanabe-Hayashi Y, Noma S, Fukuda K. Images in cardiovascular medicine. Rapid formation of left ventricular giant thrombus with Takotsubo cardiomyopathy. Circulation. 2007;115(23):e620–e1.
54. Driver K, Mangrum JM. Hybrid approaches in atrial fibrillation ablation: why, where and who? J Thorac Dis. 2015;7(2):159–64.
55. Khoynezhad A, Ellenbogen KA, Al-Atassi T, Wang PJ, Kasirajan V, Wang X, et al. Hybrid atrial fibrillation ablation: current status and a look ahead. Circ Arrhythm Electrophysiol. 2017;10(10):pii:e005263.
56. Jiang YQ, Tian Y, Zeng LJ, He SN, Zheng ZT, Shi L, et al. The safety and efficacy of hybrid ablation for the treatment of atrial fibrillation: A meta-analysis. PLoS One. 2018;13(1):e0190170.
57. Blackshear J, Odell J. Appendage obliteration to reduce stroke in cardiac surgical patients with atrial fibrillation. Ann Thorac Surg. 1996;61(2):755–9.
58. Sherwood MW, Nessel CC, Hellkamp AS, Mahaffey KW, Piccini JP, Suh EY, et al. Gastrointestinal bleeding in patients with atrial fibrillation treated with rivaroxaban or warfarin: ROCKET AF trial. J Am Coll Cardiol. 2015;66(21):2271–81.
59. Connolly SJ, Ezekowitz MD, Yusuf S, Eikelboom J, Oldgren J, Parekh A, et al. Dabigatran versus warfarin in patients with atrial fibrillation. N Engl J Med. 2009;361:1139–51.
60. Maura G, Blotiere PO, Bouillon K, Billionnet C, Ricordeau P, Alla F, et al. Comparison of the short-term risk of bleeding and arterial thromboembolic events in nonvalvular atrial fibrillation patients newly treated with dabigatran or rivaroxaban versus vitamin K antagonists: a French nationwide propensity-matched cohort study. Circulation. 2015;132(13):1252–60.
61. Reddy VY, Doshi SK, Sievert H, Buchbinder M, Neuzil P, Huber K, et al. Percutaneous left atrial appendage closure for stroke prophylaxis in patients with atrial fibrillation: 2.3-year follow-up of the PROTECT AF (watchman left atrial appendage system for embolic protection in patients with atrial fibrillation) trial. Circulation. 2013;127(6):720–9.
62. Holmes DR Jr, Kar S, Price MJ, Whisenant B, Sievert H, Doshi SK, et al. Prospective randomized evaluation of the watchman left atrial appendage closure device in patients with atrial fibrillation versus long-term warfarin therapy: the PREVAIL trial. J Am Coll Cardiol. 2014;64(1):1–12.

63. Tzikas A, Shakir S, Gafoor S, Omran H, Berti S, Santoro G, et al. Left atrial appendage occlusion for stroke prevention in atrial fibrillation: multicentre experience with the AMPLATZER cardiac plug. EuroIntervention. 2016;11(10):1170–9.
64. Lehmann LH, Riess H, Sturm I. Sickle cell disease, pulmonary hypertension, and sarcoidosis. Ann Hematol. 2008;87(7):591–2.
65. Morimoto T, Azuma A, Abe S, Usuki J, Kudoh S, Sugisaki K, et al. Epidemiology of sarcoidosis in Japan. Eur Respir J. 2008;31(2):372–9.
66. Shigemitsu H, Nagai S, Sharma OP. Pulmonary hypertension and granulomatous vasculitis in sarcoidosis. Curr Opin Pulm Med. 2007;13(5):434–8.
67. Kusa S, Miller MA, Whang W, Enomoto Y, Panizo JG, Iwasawa J, et al. Outcomes of ventricular tachycardia ablation using percutaneous left ventricular assist devices. Circ Arrhythm Electrophysiol. 2017;10(6):pii:e004717.
68. Maury P, Leobon B, Duparc A, Delay M, Galinier M. Epicardial catheter ablation of ventricular tachycardia using surgical subxyphoid approach. Europace. 2007;9(4):212–5.
69. Baughman RP, Lower EE. Six-minute walk test in managing and monitoring sarcoidosis patients. Curr Opin Pulm Med. 2007;13(5):439–44.
70. Thiene G, Corrado D, Basso C. Arrhythmogenic right ventricular cardiomyopathy/dysplasia. Orphanet J Rare Dis. 2007;2:45.
71. Anter E, Hutchinson MD, Deo R, Haqqani HM, Callans DJ, Gerstenfeld EP, et al. Surgical ablation of refractory ventricular tachycardia in patients with nonischemic cardiomyopathy. Circ Arrhythm Electrophysiol. 2011;4(4):494–500.
72. Liang JJ, Betensky BP, Muser D, Zado ES, Anter E, Desai ND, et al. Long-term outcome of surgical cryoablation for refractory ventricular tachycardia in patients with non-ischemic cardiomyopathy. Europace. 2018;20(3):e30–41.
73. Ziv O, Dizon J, Thosani A, Naka Y, Magnano AR, Garan H. Effects of left ventricular assist device therapy on ventricular arrhythmias. J Am Coll Cardiol. 2005;45(9):1428–34.
74. Shirazi JT, Lopshire JC, Gradus-Pizlo I, Hadi MA, Wozniak TC, Malik AS. Ventricular arrhythmias in patients with implanted ventricular assist devices: a contemporary review. Europace. 2013;15(1):11–7.
75. Bedi M, Kormos R, Winowich S, McNamara DM, Mathier MA, Murali S. Ventricular arrhythmias during left ventricular assist device support. Am J Cardiol. 2007;99(8):1151–3.
76. Sacher F, Reichlin T, Zado ES, Field ME, Viles-Gonzalez JF, Peichl P, et al. Characteristics of ventricular tachycardia ablation in patients with continuous flow left ventricular assist devices. Circ Arrhythm Electrophysiol. 2015;8(3):592–7.
77. Raissi Shabari F, Yousef J, Cohn W, Gregoric I, Frazier OH, Cheng J, et al. Open chest epicardial ablation of ventricular tachycardia early after left ventricular assist device implantation. J Heart Lung Transplant. 2013;32(4):S272.
78. Herweg B, Ilercil A, Kristof-Kuteyeva O, Rinde-Hoffman D, Caldeira C, Mangar D, et al. Clinical observations and outcome of ventricular tachycardia ablation in patients with left ventricular assist devices. Pacing Clin Electrophysiol. 2012;35(11):1377–83.
79. Priori SG, Wilde AA, Horie M, Cho Y, Behr ER, Berul C, et al. Executive summary: HRS/EHRA/APHRS expert consensus statement on the diagnosis and management of patients with inherited primary arrhythmia syndromes. Heart Rhythm. 2013;10(12):e85–108.
80. Nunn LM, Lambiase PD. Genetics and cardiovascular disease—causes and prevention of unexpected sudden adult death: the role of the SADS clinic. Heart. 2011;97(14):1122–7.
81. Behr ER, Dalageorgou C, Christiansen M, Syrris P, Hughes S, Tome Esteban MT, et al. Sudden arrhythmic death syndrome: familial evaluation identifies inheritable heart disease in the majority of families. Eur Heart J. 2008;29(13):1670–80.
82. Hendriks KS, Hendriks MM, Birnie E, Grosfeld FJ, Wilde AA, van den Bout J, et al. Familial disease with a risk of sudden death: a longitudinal study of the psychological consequences of predictive testing for long QT syndrome. Heart Rhythm. 2008;5(5):719–24.
83. Christiaans I, van Langen IM, Birnie E, Bonsel GJ, Wilde AA, Smets EM. Quality of life and psychological distress in hypertrophic cardiomyopathy mutation carriers: a cross-sectional cohort study. Am J Med Genet A. 2009;149A(4):602–12.

84. Adler A, Sadek MM, Chan AY, Dell E, Rutberg J, Davis D, et al. Patient outcomes from a specialized inherited arrhythmia clinic. Circ Arrhythm Electrophysiol. 2016;9(1):e003440.
85. Barry MJ, Edgman-Levitan S. Shared decision making—pinnacle of patient-centered care. N Engl J Med. 2012;366(9):780–1.
86. Charles C, Gafni A, Whelan T. Shared decision-making in the medical encounter: what does it mean? (or it takes at least two to tango). Soc Sci Med. 1997;44(5):681–92.
87. Makoul G, Clayman ML. An integrative model of shared decision making in medical encounters. Patient Educ Couns. 2006;60(3):301–12.
88. January CT, Wann LS, Alpert JS, Calkins H, Cigarroa JE, Cleveland JC Jr, et al. 2014 AHA/ACC/HRS guideline for the management of patients with atrial fibrillation: a report of the American College of Cardiology/American Heart Association task force on practice guidelines and the Heart Rhythm Society. Circulation. 2014;130(23):e199–267.
89. Masoudi FA, Calkins H, Kavinsky CJ, Drozda JP Jr, Gainsley P, Slotwiner DJ, et al. 2015 ACC/HRS/SCAI left atrial appendage occlusion device societal overview. Heart Rhythm. 2015;12(10):e122–36.
90. Al-Khatib SM, Stevenson WG, Ackerman MJ, Bryant WJ, Callans DJ, Curtis AB, et al. 2017 AHA/ACC/HRS guideline for management of patients with ventricular arrhythmias and the prevention of sudden cardiac death: executive summary: a report of the American College of Cardiology/American Heart Association Task Force on clinical practice guidelines and the Heart Rhythm Society. J Am Coll Cardiol. 2018;72(14):1677–749.
91. Bennett M, Parkash R, Nery P, Senechal M, Mondesert B, Birnie D, et al. Canadian Cardiovascular Society/Canadian Heart Rhythm Society 2016 implantable cardioverter-defibrillator guidelines. Can J Cardiol. 2017;33:174–88.
92. Lampert R, Hayes DL, Annas GJ, Farley MA, Goldstein NE, Hamilton RM, et al. HRS expert consensus statement on the management of cardiovascular implantable electronic devices (CIEDs) in patients nearing end of life or requesting withdrawal of therapy. Heart Rhythm. 2010;7(7):1008–26.
93. Stacey D, Legare F, Lewis K, Barry MJ, Bennett CL, Eden KB, et al. Decision aids for people facing health treatment or screening decisions. Cochrane Database Syst Rev. 2017;4:CD001431.
94. Legare F, Stacey D, Turcotte S, Cossi MJ, Kryworuchko J, Graham ID, et al. Interventions for improving the adoption of shared decision making by healthcare professionals. Cochrane Database Syst Rev. 2014;9:CD006732.
95. Kinnersley P, Edwards A, Hood K, Ryan R, Prout H, Cadbury N, et al. Interventions before consultations to help patients address their information needs by encouraging question asking: systematic review. BMJ. 2008;337:a485.
96. Stacey D, Kryworuchko J, Belkora J, Davison BJ, Durand MA, Eden KB, et al. Coaching and guidance with patient decision aids: a review of theoretical and empirical evidence. BMC Med Inform Decis Mak. 2013;13(Suppl 2):S11.
97. Elwyn G, O'Connor A, Stacey D, Volk R, Edwards A, Coulter A, et al. Developing a quality criteria framework for patient decision aids: online international Delphi consensus process. BMJ. 2006;333(7565):417.
98. O'Neill ES, Grande SW, Sherman A, Elwyn G, Coylewright M. Availability of patient decision aids for stroke prevention in atrial fibrillation: a systematic review. Am Heart J. 2017;191:1–11.
99. Probst MA, Noseworthy PA, Brito JP, Hess EP. Shared decision-making as the future of emergency cardiology. Can J Cardiol. 2018;34(2):117–24.
100. Jensen T, Chin J, Ashby L, Long K, Schafer J, Hakim R. Decision memo for percutaneous left atrial appendage (LAA) closure therapy (CAG-00445N). 2016.
101. Institute PCOR. $5 million award from PCORI and AHA establishes center to support better-informed AFib treatment decisions. June 18, 2018. Available from: https://www.pcori.org/news-release/5-million-award-pcori-and-aha-establishes-center-support-better-informed-afib-treatment.

102. Carroll SL, Stacey D, McGillion M, Healey JS, Foster G, Hutchings S, et al. Evaluating the feasibility of conducting a trial using a patient decision aid in implantable cardioverter defibrillator candidates: a randomized controlled feasibility trial. Pilot Feasibility Stud. 2017;3:49.
103. Jenkins A, Jones J, Mellis BK, Nuanes H, Nowels C, Varosy P, et al. Development and pilot of four decision aids for implantable cardioverter-defibrillators in different media formats. 37th annual meeting of the Society for Medical Decision Making; St Louis, Missouri. 2015.
104. Lewis KB, Birnie D, Carroll SL, Clark L, Kelly F, Gibson P, et al. User-centered development of a decision aid for patients facing implantable cardioverter-defibrillator replacement: a mixed-methods study. J Cardiovasc Nurs. 2018;33(5):481–91.
105. When to consider implantable cardioverter defibrillator (ICD) deactivation: a guide for patients and family. Toronto, ON: CorHealth; 2018.
106. Implantable cardioverter defibrillator deactivation: a guide for health care professionals. Toronto, ON: Cardiac Care Network; 2017.
107. Legare F, Stacey D, Forest PG, Coutu MF, Archambault P, Boland L, et al. Milestones, barriers and beacons: shared decision making in Canada inches ahead. Z Evid Fortbild Qual Gesundhwes. 2017;123–124:23–7.
108. Elwyn G, Scholl I, Tietbohl C, Mann M, Edwards AG, Clay C, et al. "Many miles to go …": a systematic review of the implementation of patient decision support interventions into routine clinical practice. BMC Med Inform Decis Mak. 2013;13(Suppl 2):S14.
109. Joseph-Williams N, Lloyd A, Edwards A, Stobbart L, Tomson D, Macphail S, et al. Implementing shared decision making in the NHS: lessons from the MAGIC programme. BMJ. 2017;357:j1744.
110. Friedman DJ, Al-Khatib SM. Measuring quality in electrophysiology. J Interv Card Electrophysiol. 2016;47:5–10.
111. Society CC. Quality project. Available from: http://www.ccs.ca/en/health-policy/programs-and-initiatives/quality-project. Accessed 20 July 2017.
112. Mehaffey JH, Hawkins RB, Byler M, Smith J, Kern JA, Kron I, et al. Amiodarone protocol provides cost-effective reduction in postoperative atrial fibrillation. Ann Thorac Surg. 2018;105(6):1697–702.

Patient-Centered Approach to Heart Failure Management: Transforming Care Delivery

6

Jacinthe Boulet, Nadia Giannetti, and Renzo Cecere

Clinical Vignette

Ms. V is a 62-year-old woman followed in the heart failure clinic for a non-ischemic cardiomyopathy and stage C heart failure with left ventricular ejection fraction of 25%. Her past medical history is significant for hypertension, gastroesophageal reflux disease, and a remote history of an appendectomy. She has no allergies and is a lifelong non-smoker. She drinks only one to two glasses of wine during the holidays and has never consumed any illicit drugs.

She is New York Heart Association (NYHA) Class III at baseline and is currently on optimal medical therapy as limited by heart rate and blood pressure: bisoprolol 10 mg daily, sacubitril-valsartan 97/103 mg twice daily, spironolactone 25 mg daily, and furosemide 40 mg twice daily. She is also on pantoprazole 40 mg daily as well as vitamin D 10,000 units once a week. Her baseline heart rate is 55 beats per minute so ivabradine was not considered.

She has had a negative coronary angiogram in the past. A diagnosis of idiopathic cardiomyopathy was made 5 years ago once the work-up for a potential etiology was completed, including a cardiac magnetic resonance imaging (MRI), genetic studies, and a coronary angiogram. Last year, an upgrade to cardiac resynchronization therapy defibrillator (CRT-D) from implantable cardioverter defibrillator (ICD) was done with minimal change in her symptoms.

She is socially isolated, with three cats at home. While she does have one friend who occasionally helps with groceries, she is largely independent with respect to her instrumental activities of daily living. She has had three admissions in the past year for heart failure exacerbations, including one in the context of pneumonia.

J. Boulet (✉) · N. Giannetti · R. Cecere
McGill University Health Centre, Department of Cardiology, Montreal, QC, Canada
e-mail: jacinthe.boulet@mail.mcgill.ca

© Springer Nature Switzerland AG 2019
T. Mesana (ed.), *Heart Teams for Treatment of Cardiovascular Disease*,
https://doi.org/10.1007/978-3-030-19124-5_6

Ms. V now presents to the clinic 2 weeks after her most recent hospital admission. She reports a progressive decline in her functional status over the year, with increased fatigue and occasional shortness of breath at rest. It is time to discuss further treatment directives and self-management techniques with the aim to reduce her mortality and improve her quality of life (QoL). Closer follow-up appointments are planned to minimize hospital readmissions and potentially discuss work-up for possible heart transplant or left ventricular assist device.

Now, as a health-care professional specializing in heart failure with several such patients in your practice, you ought to work with your hospital administration and cardiology department to create a multidisciplinary team (MDT) with the aim of improving patients' QoL, mortality, and hospitalization rates. You wonder about the anticipated benefits of establishing such a program as well as barriers and challenges you may encounter during this process. What would be the responsibilities of such a team? Are there any public health and economic impacts? Finally, you wonder about future directions in multidisciplinary heart failure management to adopt the most holistic approach in your clinical practice.

The Mandate of a Heart Failure Team

The burden of heart failure morbidity and mortality on patients and the health-care system in Canada is constantly growing [1]. Worldwide, heart failure with preserved and reduced ejection fraction (HFpEF and HFrEF, respectively) has reached epidemic proportions. Close to $3 billion per year from health-care costs are spent in attending to the 600,000 Canadians living with heart failure [2]. These numbers are increasing every year, and the magnitude of the epidemic has reached a level that requires action and change. Not only in Canada is heart failure becoming a major public health concern but also in the United States and worldwide, with approximately 6.5 and 23 million people, respectively, being affected by the disease [2, 3]. In the past two decades, numerous trials and meta-analyses demonstrated the importance of multidisciplinary management to decrease hospital admission rates, improve QoL, and, importantly, reduce mortality of heart failure patients both in the acute care and outpatient setting [4–6].

The mandate of a specialized and integrated heart failure team is to improve both cardiovascular outcomes and QoL through a holistic approach to a complex patient population [7]. Patient-centered care becomes crucial in the management of this syndrome, given it is a growing socioeconomic burden on public health and is the leading cause of hospital admissions in Canada [2, 8]. From the management and follow-up of chronic heart failure patients to the organization and rapid decision-making in acute cardiogenic shock, a collaborative system that connects professions has become key to transform and improve care delivery. Implementing a multidisciplinary team (MDT) would decrease mortality, facilitate transitions of care in an efficient and safe way, as well as decrease the readmission rates from all cause in heart failure patients [5, 9]. An integrated heart failure team also has the mandate of engaging patients and their families to improve patient care experience, encourage

patient self-care, and facilitate patients' comprehension of their disease through education [7–10]. Shared decision-making has become increasingly relevant with the rise of innovative therapies associated with more specialized professional expertise and procedural skills [9, 11].

Shared decision-making has been described by Elwyn and colleagues as "an approach where clinicians and patients share the best available evidence when faced with the task of making decisions, and where patients are supported to consider options, to achieve informed preferences" [9, 12]. Shared decision-making becomes even more relevant when utilizing scarce resources for patients with end-stage heart failure and who could benefit from mechanical circulatory support or heart transplant [9]. This concept reflects the importance of the patient's autonomy and must be the cornerstone of integrated specialized heart failure teams for trusting and safe relationships.

The purpose of building a specialized heart failure team also extends to education and refining evidence-based guidelines for clinicians. Multiple national guidelines already strongly recommend an MDT for the management of heart failure, and this will likely be accentuated in future guideline updates [4, 10, 13, 14]. Implementing algorithms and clinical pathways for inpatient and outpatient management will help define more clearly the role of each professional team member and will lead clinicians toward a maximized evidence-based care for heart failure patients.

Finally, the mandate of an MDT for heart failure is vast and applies to both the acute care and outpatient settings. The last few years have demonstrated the interest of clinicians to develop integrated heart failure teams and the importance of adopting a patient-centered approach for this complex population. Bringing health-care professionals together and promoting shared decision-making are the first steps toward improving cardiovascular outcomes and QoL of patients with heart failure.

Responsibilities of a Multidisciplinary Team for Heart Failure

The MDT in heart failure has become the gold standard of therapy, given the complex nature of the disease and its multisystem involvement [15]. Cardiovascular medicine is trending toward patient-centered care over disease centrism, making a wide variety of health-care professionals essential to provide best evidence practice to patients. To facilitate this, it is important to clearly define the roles and responsibilities of team members. However, there is still persistent heterogeneity regarding the nature, duration, and intensity of MDT interventions [15]. There have been numerous studies, including randomized controlled trials and meta-analyses, looking at the multidisciplinary management of heart failure patients since the 1990s [15]. Despite this, a concrete definition of such a management approach is lacking. Close collaboration between heart failure specialists, heart failure nurses, primary care physicians, cardiac surgeons, and other cardiology subspecialists is essential, along with other key members including palliative care physicians, pharmacists, social workers, physiotherapists, and dieticians (Fig. 6.1) [14, 15].

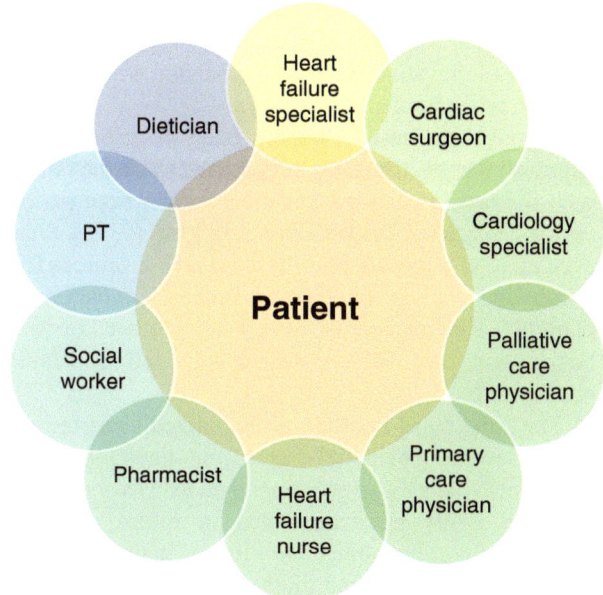

The MDT must take responsibility of the heart failure patients' care in every aspect of the disease. The team should be led by a cardiologist, specialized in heart failure. There should be clear communication and coordination between a heart failure specialist, a specialized heart failure nurse, and the patient's primary care physician. The earlier the integrated heart failure team takes ownership of patients, the most efficient are its interventions and care [15]. Heart failure specialists must be able to lead management, ensure guideline-directed medical therapy, and refer patients to other specialists, for example, electrophysiologists, endocrinologists, or nephrologists, when appropriate. The timing of referral to cardiac surgery or interventional cardiology is crucial to prevent the development of multi-organ damage and to permit the adequate use of advanced therapies [9]. Heart failure specialists, in conjunction with other members of the MDT and cardiac surgeons, must evaluate risk stratification for patients who might benefit from mechanical circulatory support and heart transplantation [9]. This is true both in the acute care setting and in specialized heart failure clinic. Given the scarcity of cardiac transplantation as a treatment resource, the role of heart failure specialists encompasses the optimal distribution of this resource, considering the principles of equity and efficiency. Collaboration between health-care professionals, including social workers and psychologists, is a must under these circumstances. Heart failure specialists also have the role of discussing prognosis as well as advanced directives and of referring patients to palliative care physicians when appropriate [16]. This can be a challenging task, as discussed later in this chapter.

Another key role of the MDT is the appropriate care of patients being discharged from the hospital and requiring close follow-up in outpatient clinics or with their

primary care physicians. One way or the other, transition of care is a critical time and should ideally be coordinated by a heart failure nurse and a heart failure specialist [17]. The target follow-up date suggested by the American College of Cardiology/American Heart Association (AHA/ACC) Guidelines is 1 week after discharge from the hospital, and, although arbitrary, it has been shown to reduce 30-day readmission rates [18, 19]. A secondary analysis of the Acute Study of Clinical Effectiveness of Nesiritide and Decompensated Heart Failure (ASCEND-HF) trial published in October 2017 in the European Journal of Heart Failure demonstrated that rehospitalization within 30 days was independently associated with increased risk for 180-day all-cause death, with a hazard ratio (HR) of 2.38 (95% confidence interval 1.93–2.94; $p < 0.001$). Thirty-three percent of all-cause readmissions occurred by day 7, and two-thirds of patients were re-hospitalized within 15 days, highlighting the importance of early follow-up.

Interventions must begin before discharge from the hospital and include optimization of guideline-directed medical therapy, ensuring dietary compliance, and facilitating cardiac rehabilitation through the help of pharmacists, dieticians, and physiotherapists. Social workers and liaison nurses can also evaluate whether patients will need help at home from local community services. Enhancing patient education prior to discharge, either through teaching by specialized heart failure nurses or instructive booklets, facilitates compliance and patients' self-management [17, 20]. Structured telephone support may also be provided by heart failure nurses or primary care physicians [17, 20]. Specialized heart failure nurses can adopt a central role in interprofessional care and have proven to enhance patient knowledge on their disease, improve self-care behaviors, and reduce heart failure readmissions [10, 21–23].

The MDT must also ensure the dissemination of medical therapy from guidelines to the bedside. In recent years, there has been emerging evidence on the roles of pharmacists, both in hospitals and in the community, as a part of multidisciplinary management of heart failure [24, 25]. The Heart Failure Society of America and the American College of Clinical Pharmacy Cardiology Practice and Research Network recommend that pharmacists be routinely involved in the care of heart failure patients to improve their clinical outcomes through rigorous drug-related problem identification and solving [26]. Pharmacists can help appropriate self-medication, improve drug safety, and introduce guideline-directed medical therapy in hospital to increase continuity in long-term use after hospital discharge [27]. They should be recruited more frequently as key members of a heart failure MDT.

The best MDT for heart failure management enhances patient-centered care and empowers patients to make appropriate decisions for their own health. Patients should receive appropriate education and reinforcement to develop the ability to self-manage their medication while monitoring their daily weights, liquid intakes, and urine outputs. Other components of self-management of heart failure include following recommendations from nurses, dieticians, and physiotherapists through a healthy diet and regular exercise [28]. Better self-care is associated with decreased hospitalization rates, improved QoL, decreased health-care costs, and, importantly, improved survival [29, 30]. The same applies to patients' caregivers, who play a

vital role in supporting heart failure patients [31]. As described in previous studies, caregivers have a positive impact on QoL, self-care, and clinical outcomes [29, 32–34]. When applicable, the MDT can thus provide a family-centered approach, optimizing heart failure education and chronic illness management of patients at home [31, 35, 36].

In summary, an MDT should be involved for all patients with heart failure and begin as early as possible after initial diagnosis. The MDT should follow patients throughout the course of their disease and respond to their changing needs. Different health-care professionals are essential for improved transitions from hospital to home, reduced hospitalizations, decreased mortality, and better QoL. Adopting a patient-centered approach is key to optimize and facilitate interventions of a dedicated heart failure team.

Benefits of a Heart Failure Team

All heart failure patients should be enrolled in a specialized and structured program to better understand their disease and make personalized choices that best suit their values and wishes. Multidisciplinary management of heart failure patients is associated with better clinical outcomes for patients and health-care professionals as well as for the health-care system [37]. The benefits of a specialized heart failure team are increasingly being recognized and introduced into numerous national guidelines, including the Canadian Cardiovascular society's latest recommendations [4]. Most importantly, there has been evidence in the literature that interprofessional and collaborative work for heart failure patients improves clinical outcomes and mortality, both in acutely ill patients and in chronic disease management [5, 6].

In a UK tertiary care center university hospital, Masters and colleagues conducted a retrospective service evaluation to assess the impacts of a specialized heart failure team intervention on treatment, hospital readmissions, and mortality [5]. The authors compared 196 patients admitted with heart failure before the introduction of a specialized team with 211 patients seen by the integrated team in its first year of operation. Five colleagues worked in collaboration for optimization of care: a cardiologist, a clinical fellow, a part-time pharmacist, and two nurses specialized in heart failure. Interventions included guideline-directed medication adjustments, regular reassessments during the patients' hospitalizations, as well as early outpatient follow-ups. The mortality in the intervention cohort was significantly reduced—both in-hospital mortality (6% vs 22%) and 1-year mortality (27% vs 43%). Additionally, there were more prescriptions of guideline-directed medical therapy as well as symptom-directed therapy in the intervention group.

In a 2017 review, Loughran and colleagues observed improved survival for patients hospitalized in a cardiovascular intensive care unit that adopted a multidisciplinary approach [38]. Similar findings were reported by Kim and colleagues in 2010 in a medical ICU population [39]. Not only in the acute care setting, but also in long-term care facilities, can multidisciplinary management reduce mortality in patients with heart failure. As early as 2004, a Journal of the American Medical

Association (JAMA) meta-analysis demonstrated that comprehensive discharge planning and better post-discharge follow-up were associated with not only reduced readmission rates but also a trend toward reduced mortality in older patients with heart failure [40]. This was reflected in the 2009 focused update of the ACC/AHA Guidelines for the Diagnosis and Management of Heart Failure in Adults [41]. Again in 2004, a systematic review published in Journal of the American College of Cardiology (JACC) recognized the impressive benefits of multidisciplinary management programs for heart failure [6]. This review, consisting of 29 randomized control trials, showed mortality reduction (risk ratio of 0.75) as well as reduction of all-cause hospitalization rates (summary risk ratio of 0.84). This corresponded to a number needed to treat of 17. Management strategies included the use of dedicated and specialized MDTs in clinic and non-clinic settings. This strategy proved superior to follow-up by regular phone calls and primary care physicians alone (RR 0.82). Regardless of the significant heterogeneity among the studies included in this review, the benefits of multidisciplinary management for heart failure patients were clear. Probably the most important benefits of a specialized heart failure team are its impact on readmission rates, length of stay, and QoL.

In the year 2013, there were 60,000 hospital visits for heart failure in Canada. This number has been steadily increasing over the past several years, with data from the Canadian Institute for Health Information (CIHI) reporting a 13% increase over the past 6 years [2]. High rehospitalization rates and early readmission to the hospital have been associated with reduced survival in patients with heart failure [6, 42–44]. While there is already good evidence for those benefits in the United States, the data is more limited in Canada, where access to the health-care system is more accessible and not restricted.

In 2005, a Montreal-based randomized trial published in the Canadian Medical Association Journal (CMAJ) demonstrated that a multidisciplinary congestive heart failure clinic compared to usual care reduces readmission rates and hospital days, as well as improves QoL [45]. This was true regardless of the patients' risk of readmission, reflecting a broader and heterogeneous heart failure population. More recently, a 2018 retrospective study in Japan with 917 patients examined 3-year hospitalization rates before and after establishing an inter-professional heart failure team [46]. Patients were identified as having heart failure when they had a serum NT-proBNP of 400 pg/ml or more. Patients diagnosed with heart failure had longer hospitalization days (median of 30 vs 18 days) compared to those without heart failure. In 303 heart failure patients followed up for 3 years after the establishment of the heart failure team, there was a marked reduction of total hospitalization days (30 vs 8 days). Multidisciplinary management reduces the length of stay and number of all-cause hospitalizations in patients with heart failure.

Adequate follow-up and support for heart failure patients is often lacking when transitioning from hospital to home [47, 48]. An innovative study out of New Hanover Regional Medical Centre focused on providing a blend of in-home and clinic-based multi-professional care involving pharmacists, community paramedics, and advanced care practitioners [24]. This approach reduced 30-day rehospitalizations from 23.5% (140 patients readmitted out of 596 patients) to 10.5% (9 patients readmitted out of

86 followed by the multidisciplinary transition of care team). Another nursing-led study in Charlotte, North Carolina, piloted a 4-week transition to care program involving 36 patients. Only 2 out of 36 patients were rehospitalized within 30 days [23]. These studies show interesting and promising results of collaborative care between primary health-care professionals to prevent rehospitalizations of patients with heart failure and ensure adequate follow-up at home after hospital discharge. As reflected in the 2016 European Society of Cardiology (ESC) guidelines for the diagnosis and treatment of acute and chronic heart failure, enrollment of patients with heart failure in a multidisciplinary-care management program is strongly encouraged (Class I, Level A of evidence) to reduce the risk of heart failure hospitalizations.

Patients with heart failure report a wide range of physical and psychosocial concerns, as well as functional limitations, that persist into day-to-day living. A patient-centered approach is vital to recognizing and suitably managing these concerns. There are several studies demonstrating the benefit of multidisciplinary care in improving QoL [26–32]. A 2017 Chinese trial involving 62 patients randomized to either multidisciplinary or standard care demonstrated significant improvements in QoL, depressive symptoms, and self-care behaviors over a 180-day period (37% vs 66%, 20% vs 61%, and 8% vs 33%, respectively, $p < 0.001$) [33]. This multidisciplinary disease management program involved discharge education, physical training, follow-up visits, and telephone calls. A large multicenter Norwegian observational study demonstrated similar improvement in QoL after 6 weeks of regular follow-up at multidisciplinary heart failure clinics [34]. Specific aspects of multidisciplinary care have also been shown to improve QoL. For instance, a meta-analysis of 16 randomized control trials demonstrated the overall effectiveness of psychosocial interventions on patient QoL [35]. However, when comparing an MDT versus physician and nurse-only delivery of care, only a trend toward benefit was observed. Additionally, the literature supports a role for exercise therapy in heart failure management. In 2009, an observational study of 116 patients studied the impact of a 4-week exercise-training program involving a physician, psychologist, dietary assistant, and sports therapist in patients with chronic heart failure [49]. In both elderly and non-elderly patients, there was an improvement in QoL after the training program and at 6 months. After 6 months, however, the elderly patients reported having an inferior QoL compared to their younger counterparts. This suggests the need for ongoing multidisciplinary support and therapy, especially in this sub-population. Since 2009, there have been several systematic reviews and meta-analyses demonstrating the benefit of exercise therapy in heart failure, as reflected in several national heart failure guidelines (CCS, AHA, and ESC).

The sections above serve to highlight the benefits of multidisciplinary management of heart failure. The simple reason behind this myriad of benefits is the observed improvement in heart failure management, in terms of pharmacological and non-pharmacological therapy. Non-pharmacological interventions for heart failure patients include appropriate use of device therapy or heart transplantation, patient self-care (fluid restriction, weight monitoring, etc.), and patient education. A 2017 study out of Melbourne piloted a general medicine multidisciplinary

heart failure program, distributing the duties of a dedicated heart failure nurse among members of a general medicine unit. Over a 6-month period, significant improvements were noted in patient education, on salt and fluid restriction, on weight monitoring, and on heart failure action plans on discharge [10]. In another instance, in a 2014 Japanese study, an inpatient multidisciplinary heart failure intervention resulted in significantly improved use of appropriate diagnostic tests, medications, cardiac rehabilitation, and patient education [50]. There is also good evidence that incorporating a pharmacist's input into a dedicated heart failure team for in-hospital as well as home management of patients' medication increases use of guideline-directed medical therapy and adherence to medication, and decreases inappropriate drug prescriptions [51–53]. Effective team communication and shared medical expertise similarly benefit patient selection for advanced therapies, such as mechanical circulatory support and heart transplantation [4, 9]. An MDT can help balance clinical factors with psychosocial factors and patient preferences, selecting those patients most likely to benefit from these therapies.

Multidisciplinary management of heart failure can also be beneficial for patients when medical or surgical options are no longer available or have been expended. In such cases, one hopes to achieve the best QoL while preparing for end-of-life. Unlike terminal cancer, there is an inherent unpredictability to the heart failure syndrome. Episodes of acutely symptomatic crises interject a varying baseline of clinical deterioration. Given this difficulty in predicting the course of end-stage heart failure, it is challenging to recognize the proper time to refer patients to a palliative care team [54]. Incorporating palliative care into the heart failure team early, while patients are hospitalized or recovering from a recent exacerbation at home, has been shown to provide several benefits [3, 55]. In the latest CCS Guideline Update on heart failure management, palliative care for heart failure was defined as a patient- and family-centered care focused on alleviating physical, psychosocial, and spiritual symptoms [4]. Importantly, the utilization of a palliative framework does not exclude the use of pharmacologic and device-based therapies intended to prolong life. The CCS guideline strongly recommends the utilization of an interdisciplinary heart failure team to ensure the optimization of available management strategies, while considering patient goals and comorbidities and avoiding treatment conflicts.

Evidence supporting early palliative care involvement in heart failure exists in both the inpatient and outpatient setting. In 2014, the PREFER randomized controlled trial demonstrated that the integration of palliative care in the home setting into standard heart failure care in patients with advanced heart failure significantly reduced symptom burden, improved their QoL, and reduced hospitalization rates [50]. A 2015 randomized controlled trial similarly demonstrated the benefits of an inpatient palliative care consult for patients hospitalized with heart failure exacerbations [56]. Finally, in the PAL-HF trial in 2017, an interdisciplinary palliative care intervention commencing in hospital and extending to the ambulatory setting resulted in clinically significant improvement in QoL, psychological symptoms, and spiritual well-being [57].

It goes without saying, although outside the scope of this book, that multiple subspecialists in cardiology are frequently part of heart failure multidisciplinary management as vital team members and contributors to patient-centered care. Their medical expertise is beneficial in various ways, such as improved patient survival, decrease hospitalizations, and improved QoL. This is well illustrated in the latest national heart failure guidelines from the ESC, AHA, and CCS.

Collaborative contributions and dedicated heart failure teams have brought numerous benefits to patient care throughout the past years. Evidenced by its positive effects on mortality, rehospitalization rates and length of stay, QoL, pharmacological and non-pharmacological management, and end-of-life care, an MDT focused on patient care, and best evidence-based practice becomes crucial for the management of heart failure.

Economic Impacts

In the 2016 Report on the health of Canadians, it was estimated that more than 2.8 billion Canadian dollars per year are spent on heart failure-associated costs [2]. In the same report, Dr. Justin Ezekowitz, director of the Heart Function Clinic at the University of Alberta, described heart failure as "the biggest driver of costs is hospitalization and emergency room visits." Similarly, in the United States, heart failure is the most expensive cause of hospital readmission, costing $32 billion annually [20, 48, 58, 59]. Given that hospital readmissions are the main driver of heart failure-associated costs, multidisciplinary management can directly decrease costs and the burden on the health-care system by significantly reducing readmission rates [60].

Different collaborative interventions in various patient populations with heart failure have been associated with lower overall costs and reduced health-care system utilization. Examples include community-based integrated systems of care for frail seniors [61–63], management of anemia in heart failure clinics [64, 65], multidisciplinary palliative care service [4], and adequate discharge planning to facilitate transition to care from hospital to home [64, 66].

In the previously mentioned 2018 study out of Japan, heart failure patients had higher total medical costs for hospitalizations compared to those without heart failure (2.42 vs 1.8 million yen). In the 303 patients followed up for 3 years by the study, with the multidisciplinary heart failure team, there were reduced medical costs of hospitalization (2.59 vs 0.76 million yen) [46]. As evidenced by a 2010 study conducted at the University Health Network in Toronto, outpatient management of heart failure patients post-hospitalization seems to be cost-effective when done in specialized multidisciplinary heart failure clinics [67]. Their cohort model was comprised of more than 16,000 patients, and the cost-effectiveness analysis was performed over a 12-year period. The heart failure clinic's incremental cost-effectiveness ratio was $18,259 for each additional life-year gained. Published in 2016, a single-centered, randomized study conducted in Spain aimed at evaluating the effects of heart failure follow-ups through telemonitoring versus routine

face-to-face encounters [68]. A total of 178 patients were enrolled in the study and the primary endpoint was nonfatal heart failure event after a follow-up period of 6 months. Per 6 months of follow-up, there was a significant mean net reduction in direct hospital costs of 3546 Euros per patient for the intervention arm. The study showed evidence that telemonitoring of heart failure patients may lead to lower costs as well as better clinical outcomes ([HR] for the primary endpoint was 0.35 (95% confidence interval [CI], 0.20–0.59; p value <0.001)).

In the case of end-stage heart failure, advanced therapeutic options can put a financial strain on the health-care system unless an organized and efficient care plan is put in place. In a prospective cohort study performed in 2008, Murray and colleagues identified that multidisciplinary management versus a single-discipline service, i.e., cardiac surgery can benefit patients following left ventricular assist device therapy with reduced length of stay in the hospital as well as lower costs [66]. In this study, patients were managed by a heart failure specialist and cardiothoracic surgeon, with patient and family education initiated in the intensive care unit. Other health-care professionals such as physiotherapists and occupational therapists began their assessment in the intensive care unit as well, and patients were referred to cardiac rehabilitation center upon discharge. There was a 78% reduction of total costs observed for patients managed by the MDT compared with the cardiac surgery team alone. Even in patients with end-stage heart failure who are not candidates for advanced therapeutic options such as mechanical circulatory support or cardiac transplantation, multidisciplinary management involving a palliative care team helps to avoid the inappropriate escalation of care and high costs commonly seen at the end of life [69].

Whether in the acute setting of an intensive care unit or in chronic management of the disease in dedicated clinics, introducing a specialized heart failure team offers significant reductions in total costs, which are mainly driven by hospital readmission rates. Collaborative work of various health-care professionals for the management of heart failure should be more strongly encouraged and instituted to decrease the financial burden of the disease on the health-care system.

Challenges and Barriers

Adopting a holistic approach to heart failure through collaborative work has many beneficial impacts on delivery of care. Despite all of the advantages of multidisciplinary management, some challenges exist that hinder the implementation of such a practice.

Efficient teamwork that takes advantage of the clinical expertise of different health-care professionals has been shown to improve the quality of care for patients with heart failure. Some barriers to well-organized and productive collaboration include incompatible leadership, inappropriate interactions and communication within the team, resistance to change, heavy workload, and fatigue [11, 70, 71]. In February 2018, an Iranian nurse-lead qualitative content analysis aimed to assess the barriers to effectiveness of teamwork in a total of 58 members working with

heart failure patients [11]. Those members included staff physicians, patients, physiotherapists, nutritionists, nursing managers, and staff nurses. Most participants in this study identified disease centrism (instead of patient centrism), wide hierarchies, and cultural diversity as impediments to teamwork in caring for heart failure patients. Other authors have identified communication challenges and differences in methodologies as major barriers that hamper the institution of MDTs [72]. Eliminating those barriers and creating favorable relationships is vital in order to provide safer management to patients and better quality of care [71].

An additional limitation to fully implement interdisciplinary team approaches is how "schools fail to better prepare their students and trainees with skills that allow them to work in or lead teams." An article published in CJC in 2014 by Clark and colleagues described strengths and weaknesses of different team models, emphasizing the training program implemented by the Alberta Heart Failure Etiology and Analysis Research Team (HEART) [72]. The Alberta HEART training program for research in heart failure with preserve ejection fraction (STEADI HF) was built to fully prepare trainees for transdisciplinary work. This program helps young investigators become accomplished leaders of interprofessional teams focused on understanding heart failure with preserved ejection fraction. In short, on top of their own expertise, members enrolled in the program must familiarize themselves with skills that are distinct from their own, promoting interdisciplinary partnership. This type of training for young scientific researchers could easily be applicable to the training of health-care professionals to meet the increasing need of multidisciplinary work in heart failure management.

The difficulty of properly establishing an interprofessional framework to improve the management of heart failure toward better patient-centered care also derives from institutional and governmental limitations. Despite the proven benefits on patient and system outcomes of multidisciplinary disease management, this care model is not easily implemented in health-care centers where skilled heart failure physicians or specialized heart failure nurses are not always present [73]. There is great variability in access to care as well as in distribution of resources between institutions, such as super hospitals and tertiary care centers, community hospitals, and dedicated heart institutes [73]. Also, compared to institutions such as the Ottawa Heart Institute or the Montreal Heart Institute in Canada, distribution of resources becomes a matter of potential struggle in tertiary care centers where subspecialties compete for monitored intensive care beds, either in the CCU, CVICU, or ICU. As well, financial disparities are a major contributor to the difficulty to translate clinical advances and ensure equal access to optimal heart failure care, which includes interprofessional decision-making [73]. Consequently, outcomes from randomized controlled trials and guideline-based recommendations may not necessarily reflect real-world practice, especially in resource-limited settings [10, 73]. In summary, we need simple, uniform, and easily replicable approaches to enable the implementation of best-practice guidelines. It is particularly important that these approaches are accessible by teams not only operating in tertiary care centers or dedicated cardiac hospitals but also in community centers and outpatient clinics as well.

The unpredictable course and prognosis of heart failure makes it challenging for health-care professionals to best care for patients at the end of life. Additionally, patients' own understanding of their disease and the diversity of their values and cultural backgrounds also complicate discussion about goals of care and decisions on when to aim for comfort measures and QoL rather than quantity of life and advanced therapies. As a result, only 20% of patients with heart failure have documented goals of care through advance directives certification [74]. Unlike cancer, heart failure is characterized by alternating periods of exacerbations and remissions, during which it is difficult to appropriately assess the course of the disease. As described previously, involving palliative care in the multidisciplinary management of heart failure patients reduces symptom burden, improves QoL, and reduces hospitalization rates [4, 50, 55, 56]. Patients and families are often unwilling to hear about limited life expectancy, and physicians often defer palliative care referral and discussion of advance directives [54, 55, 74]. A common issue in a way unique to the heart failure population is ICD deactivation at the end of life [16]. To prevent unnecessary shock and improve QoL, heart failure specialists must provide appropriate patient education through enhanced communication, potentially in collaboration with palliative care physicians and nurses.

Broadly validated and widely used risk stratification models such as the Seattle Heart Failure Model and the Heart Failure Survival Score have been shown to have excellent prognostic value and may be of help to guide shared decision-making with heart failure patients [9]. This is also true for patients with end-staged heart failure who are eligible for mechanical circulatory support as well as cardiac transplantation. Despite prediction tools and heart failure specialists' experience, management of advanced heart failure remains imprecise and challenging. A collaborative approach between specialized health-care professionals and patients facilitates the development of a comprehensive care plan for patients, as well as the distribution of available resources, but many important barriers continue to remain in place [9, 55].

Conclusion: The Future of Multidisciplinary Teams

The future of heart failure care is promising and exciting, as the management of the disease is shifting toward a more personalized and collaborative approach. MDTs are becoming increasingly important as the burden of the disease is growing. In clinical and basic science research, there is continued interest in discovering new disease targets and management strategies to optimize patient outcomes and provide equal access to best-evidence practice. The collaboration of a diverse group of health-care professionals will facilitate the exchange of ideas across a variety of clinical expertise and training backgrounds. Together, members of the MDT can generate unique and innovative ideas for the prevention and treatment of heart failure.

Potential upcoming personalized strategies in heart failure include remote monitoring through implantable electronic devices (e.g., CardioMEMS), biomarker-guided management (e.g., natriuretic peptides), innovative regeneration and repair

of heart function (e.g., tissue engineering), as well as genetic targets for cardiomyopathies [73]. In the next few years, several anticipated clinical trials might positively impact heart failure management. Those include COMMANDER HF looking at cardiovascular outcomes with rivaroxaban in heart failure, VICTORIA assessing potential impacts on cardiovascular death and heart failure hospitalization of vericiguat in heart failure with reduced ejection fraction, GALACTIC-HF looking at the same outcomes as the VICTORIA trial for the cardiac-specific myosin activator omecamtiv mecarbil, DAPA-HF-EMPEROR evaluating the effects of dapagliflozin and empagliflozin on heart failure patients, and finally PARAGON-HF comparing global outcomes between angiotensin receptor-neprilysin inhibitor (ARNi) and angiotensin receptor blockers (ARB) in heart failure with preserved ejection fraction [73]. If and when these trials are incorporated into guideline-based therapies, it will be multidisciplinary team members who will assess therapy candidacy, prescribe, monitor, and advise patients, providing personalized heart failure management.

The MDT is best suited to recognize the needs of heart failure patients while having the know-how to appropriately manage them, thereby optimizing outcomes. With ever-increasing disease burden, often without proportional increases in funding, more research is urgently required to identify which MDT interventions are most effective, efficient, and scalable. It is important to look past short-term costs, as a successful MDT heart failure program results in significant mortality, symptomatic, and economic benefits. With ongoing research, the potential of the MDT is far from exhausted. Indeed, the MDT approach to heart failure may serve as an exemplar for other disease states and other specialties.

References

1. Virani SA, Bains M, Code J, Ducharme A, Harkness K, Howlett JG, et al. The need for heart failure advocacy in Canada. Can J Cardiol. 2017;33(11):1450–4.
2. Heart and Stroke Foundation. 2016 report on the health of Canadians: the burden of heart failure. Available at: www.heartandstroke.ca. Accessed 30 Apr 2018.
3. Benjamin EJ, Blaha MJ, Chiuve SE, Cushman M, Das SR, Deo R, et al. Heart disease and stroke statistics—2017 update: a report from the American Heart Association. Circulation. 2017;135(10):e146–603.
4. Ezekowitz JA, O'Meara E, McDonald MA, Abrams H, Chan M, Ducharme A, et al. 2017 comprehensive update of the Canadian Cardiovascular Society guidelines for the management of heart failure. Can J Cardiol. 2017;33(11):1342–433.
5. Masters J, Morton G, Anton I, Szymanski J, Greenwood E, Grogono J, et al. Specialist intervention is associated with improved patient outcomes in patients with decompensated heart failure: evaluation of the impact of a multidisciplinary inpatient heart failure team. Open Heart. 2017;4(1):e000547.
6. McAlister FA, Stewart S, Ferrua S, McMurray JJ. Multidisciplinary strategies for the management of heart failure patients at high risk for admission: a systematic review of randomized trials. J Am Coll Cardiol. 2004;44(4):810–9.
7. Zierler BK, Abu-Rish Blakeney E, O'Brien KD, Teams IHF. An interprofessional collaborative practice approach to transform heart failure care: an overview. J Interprof Care. 2018;32(3):378–81.

8. Dunlay SM, Roger VL. Understanding the epidemic of heart failure: past, present, and future. Curr Heart Fail Rep. 2014;11(4):404–15.
9. Vucicevic D, Honoris L, Raia F, Deng M. Current indications for transplantation: stratification of severe heart failure and shared decision-making. Ann Cardiothorac Surg. 2018;7(1):56–66.
10. Wahbi-Izzettin O, Hopper I, Ritchie E, Nagalingam V, Aung AK. United we stand, divided we conquer: pilot study of multidisciplinary general medicine heart failure care program. Intern Med J. 2018;48(2):178–83.
11. Khoshab H, Nouhi E, Tirgari B, Ahmadi F. Invisible cobwebs in teamwork-impediments to the care of patients with heart failure: a qualitative study. Int J Health Plann Manag. 2018;33(2):e663–73.
12. Elwyn G, Frosch D, Thomson R, Joseph-Williams N, Lloyd A, Kinnersley P, et al. Shared decision making: a model for clinical practice. J Gen Intern Med. 2012;27(10):1361–7.
13. Yancy CW, Jessup M, Bozkurt B, Butler J, Casey DE, Colvin MM, et al. 2017 ACC/AHA/HFSA focused update of the 2013 ACCF/AHA guideline for the management of Heart Failure: a report of the American College of Cardiology/American Heart Association Task Force on clinical practice guidelines and the Heart Failure Society of America. Circulation. 2017;36(6):e137–61.
14. Ponikowski P, Voors AA, Anker SD, Bueno H, Cleland JGF, Coats AJS, et al. 2016 ESC guidelines for the diagnosis and treatment of acute and chronic heart failure. The Task Force for the diagnosis and treatment of acute and chronic heart failure of the European Society of Cardiology (ESC) developed with the special contribution of the Heart Failure Association (HFA) of the ESC. Eur Heart J. 2016;37(27):2129–200.
15. Morton G, Masters J, Cowburn PJ. Multidisciplinary team approach to heart failure management. Heart. 2017;23:23.
16. You JJ, Aleksova N, Ducharme A, MacIver J, Mielniczuk L, Fowler RA, et al. Barriers to goals of care discussions with patients who have advanced heart failure: results of a multicenter survey of hospital-based cardiology clinicians. J Card Fail. 2017;23(11):786–93.
17. Edelmann F, Knosalla C, Morike K, Muth C, Prien P, Stork S. Chronic heart failure. Dtsch Arztebl Int. 2018;115(8):124–30.
18. Hernandez AF, Greiner MA, Fonarow GC, Hammill BG, Heidenreich PA, Yancy CW, et al. Relationship between early physician follow-up and 30-day readmission among Medicare beneficiaries hospitalized for heart failure. JAMA. 2010;303(17):1716–22.
19. Yancy CW, Jessup M, Bozkurt B, Butler J, Casey DE Jr, Drazner MH, et al. 2013 ACCF/AHA guideline for the management of heart failure: a report of the American College of Cardiology Foundation/American Heart Association Task Force on Practice Guidelines. J Am Coll Cardiol. 2013;62(16):e147–239.
20. Nazir A, Smucker WD. Heart failure in post-acute and long-term care: evidence and strategies to improve transitions, clinical care, and quality of life. J Am Med Dir Assoc. 2015;16(10):825–31.
21. Manning S. Bridging the gap between hospital and home: a new model of care for reducing readmission rates in chronic heart failure. J Cardiovasc Nurs. 2011;26(5):368–76.
22. Anderson JH. Nursing presence in a community heart failure program. Nurs Pract. 2007;32(10):14–21.
23. Whitaker-Brown CD, Woods SJ, Cornelius JB, Southard E, Gulati SK. Improving quality of life and decreasing readmissions in heart failure patients in a multidisciplinary transition-to-care clinic. Heart Lung. 2017;46(2):79–84.
24. Boykin A, Wright D, Stevens L, Gardner L. Interprofessional care collaboration for patients with heart failure. Am J Health Syst Pharm. 2018;75(1):e45–9.
25. Anderson SL, Marrs JC. A review of the role of the pharmacist in heart failure transition of care. Adv Ther. 2018;35(3):311–23.
26. Milfred-Laforest SK, Chow SL, Didomenico RJ, Dracup K, Ensor CR, Gattis-Stough W, et al. Clinical pharmacy services in heart failure: an opinion paper from the Heart Failure Society of America and American College of Clinical Pharmacy Cardiology Practice and Research Network. J Card Fail. 2013;19(5):354–69.

27. Gattis WA, O'Connor CM. Predischarge initiation of carvedilol in patients hospitalized for decompensated heart failure. Am J Cardiol. 2004;93(9A):74B–6.
28. Jaarsma T, Beattie JM, Ryder M, Rutten FH, McDonagh T, Mohacsi P, et al. Palliative care in heart failure: a position statement from the palliative care workshop of the Heart Failure Association of the European Society of Cardiology. Eur J Heart Fail. 2009;11(5):433–43.
29. Clark AM, Spaling M, Harkness K, Spiers J, Strachan PH, Thompson DR, et al. Determinants of effective heart failure self-care: a systematic review of patients' and caregivers' perceptions. Heart. 2014;100(9):716–21.
30. Riegel B, Moser DK, Anker SD, Appel LJ, Dunbar SB, Grady KL, et al. State of the science: promoting self-care in persons with heart failure: a scientific statement from the American Heart Association. Circulation. 2009;120(12):1141–63.
31. Nimmon L, Bates J, Kimel G, Lingard L. Patients with heart failure and their partners with chronic illness: interdependence in multiple dimensions of time. J Multidiscip Healthc. 2018;11:175–86.
32. Zhang KM, Dindoff K, Arnold JMO, Lane J, Swartzman LC. What matters to patients with heart failure? The influence of non-health-related goals on patient adherence to self-care management. Patient Educ Couns. 2015;98(8):927–34.
33. Heo S, Lennie TA, Moser DK, Kennedy RL. Types of social support and their relationships to physical and depressive symptoms and health-related quality of life in patients with heart failure. Heart Lung. 2014;43(4):299–305.
34. Molloy GJ, Johnston DW, Witham MD. Family caregiving and congestive heart failure. Review and analysis. Eur J Heart Fail. 2005;7(4):592–603.
35. Ågren S, Evangelista L, Strömberg A. Do partners of patients with chronic heart failure experience caregiver burden? Eur J Cardiovasc Nurs. 2010;9(4):254–62.
36. Dunbar SB, Clark PC, Quinn C, Gary RA, Kaslow NJ. Family influences on heart failure self-care and outcomes. J Cardiovasc Nurs. 2008;23(3):258–65.
37. Wijeysundera HC, Trubiani G, Wang X, Mitsakakis N, Austin PC, Ko DT, et al. A population-based study to evaluate the effectiveness of multidisciplinary heart failure clinics and identify important service components. Circ Heart Fail. 2013;6(1):68–75.
38. Loughran J, Puthawala T, Sutton BS, Brown LE, Pronovost PJ, DeFilippis AP. The cardiovascular intensive care unit-an evolving model for health care delivery. J Intensive Care Med. 2017;32(2):116–23.
39. Kim MM, Barnato AE, Angus DC, Fleisher LA, Kahn JM. The effect of multidisciplinary care teams on intensive care unit mortality. Arch Intern Med. 2010;170(4):369–76.
40. Phillips CO, Wright SM, Kern DE, Singa RM, Shepperd S, Rubin HR. Comprehensive discharge planning with postdischarge support for older patients with congestive heart failure: a meta-analysis. JAMA. 2004;291(11):1358–67.
41. Hunt SA, Abraham WT, Chin MH, Feldman AM, Francis GS, Ganiats TG, et al. 2009 focused update incorporated into the ACC/AHA 2005 guidelines for the diagnosis and management of heart failure in adults. A report of the American College of Cardiology Foundation/American Heart Association task force on practice guidelines developed in collaboration with the International Society for Heart and Lung Transplantation. J Am Coll Cardiol. 2009;53(15):e1–90.
42. Fudim M, O'Connor CM, Dunning A, Ambrosy AP, Armstrong PW, Coles A, et al. Aetiology, timing and clinical predictors of early vs. late readmission following index hospitalization for acute heart failure: insights from ASCEND-HF. Eur J Heart Fail. 2018;20(2):304–14.
43. Arundel C, Lam PH, Khosla R, Blackman MR, Fonarow GC, Morgan C, et al. Association of 30-day all-cause readmission with long-term outcomes in hospitalized older Medicare beneficiaries with heart failure. Am J Med. 2016;129(11):1178–84.
44. Setoguchi S, Stevenson LW, Schneeweiss S. Repeated hospitalizations predict mortality in the community population with heart failure. Am Heart J. 2007;154(2):260–6.
45. Ducharme A, Doyon O, White M, Rouleau JL, Brophy JM. Impact of care at a multidisciplinary congestive heart failure clinic: a randomized trial. CMAJ. 2005;173(1):40–5.

46. Kitagawa T, Oda N, Mizukawa M, Hidaka T, Naka M, Nakayama S, et al. Hospitalization and medical cost of patients with elevated serum N-terminal pro-brain natriuretic peptide levels. PLoS One. 2018;13(1):e0190979.
47. Naylor MD, Aiken LH, Kurtzman ET, Olds DM, Hirschman KB. The importance of transitional care in achieving health reform. Health Aff (Millwood). 2011;30(4):746–54.
48. Stamp KD, Machado MA, Allen NA. Transitional care programs improve outcomes for heart failure patients: an integrative review. J Cardiovasc Nurs. 2014;29(2):140–54.
49. Miche E, Roelleke E, Zoller B, Wirtz U, Schneider M, Huerst M, et al. A longitudinal study of quality of life in patients with chronic heart failure following an exercise training program. Eur J Cardiovasc Nurs. 2009;8(4):281–7.
50. Brannstrom M, Boman K. Effects of person-centred and integrated chronic heart failure and palliative home care. PREFER: a randomized controlled study. Eur J Heart Fail. 2014;16(10):1142–51.
51. Milfred-LaForest SK, Gee JA, Pugacz AM, Pina IL, Hoover DM, Wenzell RC, et al. Heart failure transitions of care: a pharmacist-led post-discharge pilot experience. Prog Cardiovasc Dis. 2017;60(2):249–58.
52. Suzuki M, Matsue Y, Izumi S, Kimura A, Hashimoto T, Otomo K, et al. Pharmacist-led intervention in the multidisciplinary team approach optimizes heart failure medication. Heart Vessel. 2017;04:04.
53. Parajuli DR, Franzon J, McKinnon RA, Shakib S, Clark RA. Role of the pharmacist for improving self-care and outcomes in heart failure. Curr Heart Fail Rep. 2017;14(2):78–86.
54. Kurozumi Y, Oishi S, Sugano Y, Sakashita A, Kotooka N, Suzuki M, et al. Design of a nationwide survey on palliative care for end-stage heart failure in Japan. J Cardiol. 2018;71(2):202–11.
55. Ryder M, Beattie JM, O'Hanlon R, McDonald K. Multidsciplinary heart failure management and end of life care. Curr Opin Support Palliat Care. 2011;5(4):317–21.
56. Sidebottom AC, Jorgenson A, Richards H, Kirven J, Sillah A. Inpatient palliative care for patients with acute heart failure: outcomes from a randomized trial. J Palliat Med. 2015;18(2):134–42.
57. Rogers JG, Patel CB, Mentz RJ, Granger BB, Steinhauser KE, Fiuzat M, et al. Palliative care in heart failure: the PAL-HF randomized, controlled clinical trial. J Am Coll Cardiol. 2017;70(3):331–41.
58. Heidenreich PA, Trogdon JG, Khavjou OA, Butler J, Dracup K, Ezekowitz MD, et al. Forecasting the future of cardiovascular disease in the United States. A policy statement from the American Heart Association. Circulation. 2011;123(8):933–44.
59. Kociol RD, Peterson ED, Hammill BG, Flynn KE, Heidenreich PA, Piña IL, et al. National survey of hospital strategies to reduce heart failure readmissions: findings from the Get With the Guidelines-Heart Failure registry. Circ Heart Fail. 2012;5(6):680–7.
60. Moertl D, Steiner S, Coyle D, Berger R. Cost-utility analysis of nt-probnp-guided multidisciplinary care in chronic heart failure. Int J Technol Assess Health Care. 2013;29(1):3–11.
61. McDonald KM, Sundaram V, Bravata DM, Lewis R, Lin N, Kraft SA, et al. Closing the quality gap: a critical analysis of quality improvement strategies (vol 7: care coordination). Rockville: AHRQ Technical Reviews. Agency for Healthcare Research and Quality (US); 2007. Report No.: 04(07)-0051-7.
62. Mackie S, Darvill A. Factors enabling implementation of integrated health and social care: a systematic review. Br J Community Nurs. 2016;21(2):82–7.
63. Del Sindaco D, Pulignano G, Minardi G, Apostoli A, Guerrieri L, Rotoloni M, et al. Two-year outcome of a prospective, controlled study of a disease management programme for elderly patients with heart failure. J Cardiovasc Med (Hagerstown). 2007;8(5):324–9.
64. Davis JD, Olsen MA, Bommarito K, LaRue SJ, Saeed M, Rich MW, et al. All-payer analysis of heart failure hospitalization 30-day readmission: comorbidities matter. Am J Med. 2017;130(1):93.e9–28.
65. Nordyke RJ, Kim JJ, Goldberg GA, Vendiola R, Batra D, McCamish M, et al. Impact of anemia on hospitalization time, charges, and mortality in patients with heart failure. Value Health. 2004;7(4):464–71.

66. Murray MA, Osaki S, Edwards NM, Johnson MR, Bobadilla JL, Gordon EA, et al. Multidisciplinary approach decreases length of stay and reduces cost for ventricular assist device therapy. Interact Cardiovasc Thorac Surg. 2009;8(1):84–8.
67. Wijeysundera HC, Machado M, Wang X, Van Der Velde G, Sikich N, Witteman W, et al. Cost-effectiveness of specialized multidisciplinary heart failure clinics in Ontario, Canada. Value Health. 2010;13(8):915–21.
68. Comin-Colet J, Enjuanes C, Verdu-Rotellar JM, Linas A, Ruiz-Rodriguez P, Gonzalez-Robledo G, et al. Impact on clinical events and healthcare costs of adding telemedicine to multidisciplinary disease management programmes for heart failure: results of a randomized controlled trial. J Telemed Telecare. 2016;22(5):282–95.
69. Brian Cassel J, Kerr KM, McClish DK, Skoro N, Johnson S, Wanke C, et al. Effect of a home-based palliative care program on healthcare use and costs. J Am Geriatr Soc. 2016;64(11):2288–95.
70. O'Daniel M, Rosenstein AH. Professional communication and team collaboration. In: Hughes RG, editor. Patient safety and quality: an evidence-based handbook for nurses. Rockville: Advances in Patient Safety; 2008.
71. Weller J, Boyd M, Cumin D. Teams, tribes and patient safety: overcoming barriers to effective teamwork in healthcare. Postgrad Med J. 2014;90(1061):149–54.
72. Clark AM, Narine KA, Hsu ZY, Wiens KS, Anderson TJ, Dyck JR, et al. Preparing today's cardiovascular trainees to meet the challenges of tomorrow: team research and interdisciplinary training. Can J Cardiol. 2014;30(6):683–6.
73. McDonald MA, Ashley EA, Fedak PWM, Hawkins N, Januzzi JL, McMurray JJV, et al. Mind the gap: current challenges and future state of heart failure care. Can J Cardiol. 2017;33(11):1434–49.
74. Gasper AM, Magdic K, Ren D, Fennimore L. Development of a home health-based palliative care program for patients with heart failure. Home Healthc Now. 2018;36(2):84–92.

Heart Teams for Women's Heart Health: Advancing Cardiovascular Prevention and Care for Women

Thais Coutinho

Introduction

Heart Teams consist of multidisciplinary teams of healthcare providers working collaboratively in the decision-making process to determine the best management strategies for individual patients. Through sharing of expertise, implementation of best practices, and provision of an open forum for discussion of systems' strengths and weaknesses, Heart Teams advance patient care and create a platform for collaboration and innovation.

Coronary revascularization, cardiac transplantation, and transcatheter aortic valve replacement (TAVR) have been the most common subjects of Heart Teams. The need for a Coronary Heart Team has been emphasized in Canadian [1], American [2, 3], and European [4] practice guidelines. Similarly, Canadian guidelines recommend a multidisciplinary consensus from Heart Team members in TAVR decisions [5]. Outside of the cardiology realm, the effects of multidisciplinary teams have been well documented in the field of oncology. Such an approach has led to improvements in communication, continuity of care, time to treatment initiation, guideline adherence, and professional satisfaction [6, 7]. In specific cancers, improved survival outcomes have also been observed. For example, among women with breast cancer, survival improved by a relative 11% with a multidisciplinary approach, when compared to usual care [8]. Therefore, as healthcare providers face an increase in medical complexity, multidisciplinary teams have significant potential to increase the efficacy and efficiency of care.

T. Coutinho (✉)
University of Ottawa Heart Institute, Department of Cardiology, Ottawa, ON, Canada
e-mail: tcoutinho@ottawaheart.ca

© Springer Nature Switzerland AG 2019
T. Mesana (ed.), *Heart Teams for Treatment of Cardiovascular Disease*,
https://doi.org/10.1007/978-3-030-19124-5_7

The Need for a Women's Heart Health Team in Healthcare Institutions

The issues affecting the field of women's cardiovascular health are distinctly different than those being addressed by current coronary revascularization, TAVR, and cardiac transplantation Heart Teams. Providers working in cardiovascular medicine are faced with a relative paucity of scientific data to drive clinical decisions in women: as of 2018, two-thirds of clinical cardiovascular research have focused on men [9]. Further, levels of awareness about specific cardiovascular issues affecting women are low in the community [10] and among healthcare providers [11]. This is partially due to the fact that, despite advances in knowledge in the past few decades, there is no specific curriculum dedicated to women's cardiovascular health at undergraduate, graduate, or postgraduate levels. Moreover, cardiovascular practice guidelines often refer to women as "special populations," despite the fact that there are nearly as many women as men in the world and cardiovascular diseases are the No. 1 killers of women worldwide. By transmitting such a message of peripheralization, women's cardiovascular health is marginalized. Collectively, these issues lead to significant knowledge and practice gaps that ultimately undermine a woman's cardiovascular care and health. Therefore, in order to overcome existing obstacles and improve research, knowledge, and practice of cardiovascular health in women, institutions need to bring these issues into the core of their priorities and strategic planning. By centralizing women's cardiovascular health issues, healthcare centers will have the ability to change institutional culture, promote dissemination of knowledge, motivate engagement, develop necessary internal policies, and ultimately improve the quality and efficiency of cardiovascular prevention and care for women.

A simplified process guiding the development of a Women's Heart Health Team is depicted in Fig. 7.1. The first step toward assimilating the need for a Women's Heart Health Team is to understand that well-known sex and gender differences exist in the pathophysiology, clinical manifestations, efficacy of diagnostic tests, availability and efficacy of treatments, and clinical outcomes of cardiovascular diseases [12–28]. Furthermore, some cardiovascular disorders are either unique to women [29, 30] or more prevalent in women than men [31–33]. Knowledge of such differences, coupled with understanding of each institution's strengths, weaknesses, and gaps in knowledge and care in the field of women's cardiovascular health, will help healthcare institutions develop the necessary membership and strategic planning for their Women's Heart Health Teams.

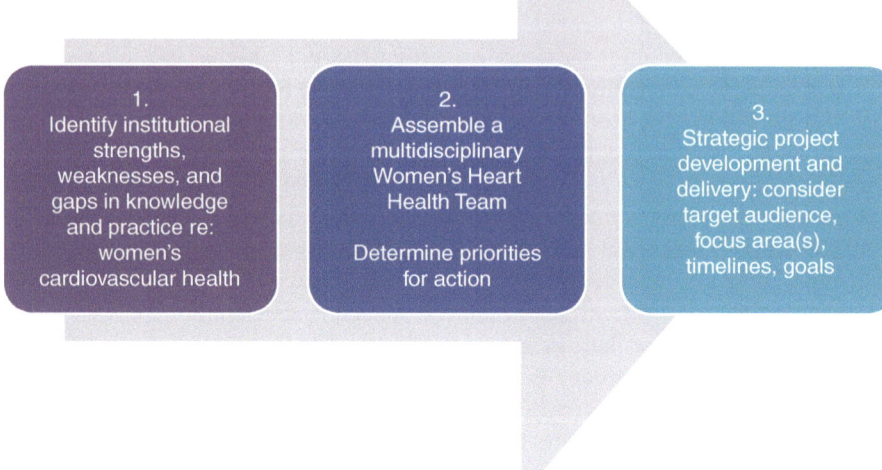

Fig. 7.1 Steps for the creation of a Women's Heart Health Team at healthcare institutions. The first step is to understand institutional culture regarding women's cardiovascular health—what are the gaps in knowledge and care among staff? What are the institution's strengths and weaknesses in the field of women's cardiovascular health? This reflection will lead to establishing the necessary membership of the Women's Heart Health Team, in addition to the priorities for action and strategic planning. Once the team is established, projects and timelines can be developed, taking into account target audiences, goals, and area(s) of focus (e.g., clinical care, education, research, or advocacy)

Sex and Gender Differences in Coronary Heart Disease: Highlighting Existing Knowledge that Supports a Dedicated Women's Heart Health Team

Gaps in knowledge about the unique aspects of cardiovascular disease in women lead to suboptimal care. As such, a Women's Heart Health Team would be in prime position to eliminate knowledge and care gaps at the institutional level. Since coronary heart disease (CHD) is the most common reason for cardiovascular outpatient and inpatient services in most institutions, it will be used here as a "model" to illustrate the potential scope of a Women's Heart Health Team. When it comes to CHD, applying the same diagnostic and treatment strategies to men and women may lead to several cases of missed diagnoses and inappropriate treatments in women, highlighting a perfect scenario for institutional action.

CHD Risk Factors

Commonly used cardiovascular risk scores tend to underestimate future cardiovascular risk in women, especially younger women [34]. The main problem with the short-term risk estimation provided by conventional risk scores is that women traditionally have a lower short-term cardiovascular risk but a higher lifetime risk [34]. Further, although conventional risk factors are the same for men and women, several risk factors will have a stronger contribution to the development of CHD in women than in men. For example, hypertension has a stronger population-attributable risk for myocardial infarction [35], stroke [36], heart failure [37], target-organ damage [38], and death [39] in women than in men. Similarly, diabetes increases the risk for CHD by three- to sevenfold in women, compared to two- to threefold in men [40]; and smoking is also a more potent risk factor for women [41]. In addition, women are exposed to a number of sex-specific risk factors that are not incorporated in conventional cardiovascular risk score estimations. For example, women with a history of hypertensive disorders of pregnancy have a 3.7-fold increase in the risk of chronic hypertension, a 2.5-fold increase in the risk of myocardial infarction, four times higher risk of heart failure, 81% higher risk of stroke, and a 2.2-fold increase in the risk of cardiovascular death compared to women with normotensive pregnancies (Fig. 7.2) [29]. Inflammatory autoimmune conditions such as rheumatoid

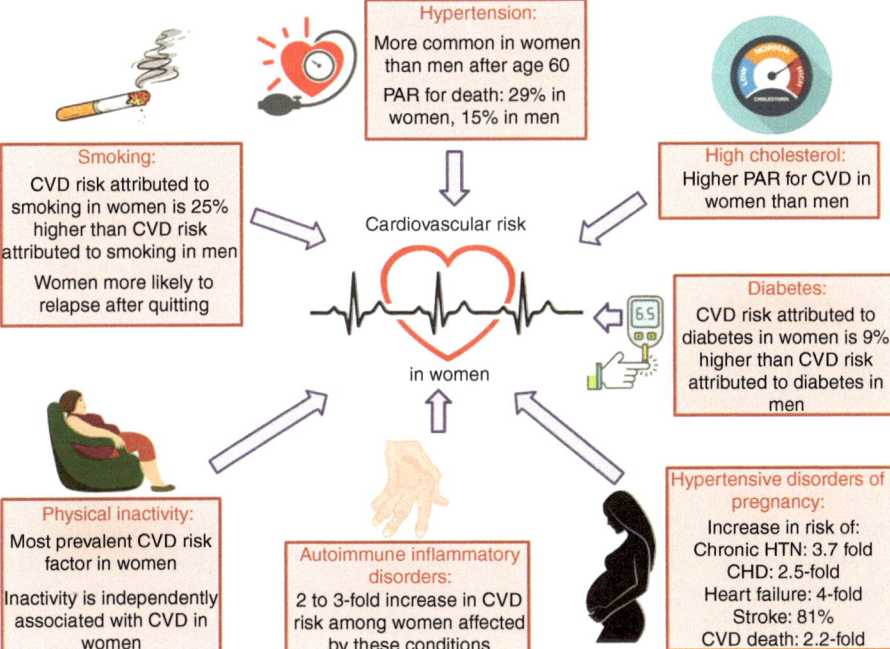

Fig. 7.2 Specific aspects of cardiovascular risk in women. Conventional risk factors are typically more ominous in women. In addition, women have nonconventional risk factors, such as hypertensive disorders of pregnancy or autoimmune inflammatory conditions (predominantly affecting women), which are not incorporated in traditional risk scores, but need to be considered by clinicians. CHD, coronary heart disease; CVD, cardiovascular disease; HTN, hypertension; PAR, population-attributable risk

arthritis and systemic lupus erythematosus also increase one's cardiovascular risk [42]. While these conditions can be present in men or women, women are much more commonly affected than men. Clinicians need to be knowledgeable about these unique aspects of cardiovascular risk in women in order to provide the best possible preventative strategies.

CHD Pathophysiology

Among women who have a myocardial infarction with angiographically "normal" coronary arteries, 38% had evidence of plaque disruption (rupture or ulceration) on intravascular ultrasound [43]. Women appear to have more diffuse atherosclerosis, less luminal stenosis, higher incidence of endothelial dysfunction, and a higher prevalence of microvascular dysfunction than men [44]. Furthermore, among people presenting to the Emergency Department with chest pain but rule out for myocardial infarction, women are four times more likely than men to have microvascular dysfunction [45]; and such a condition would not be diagnosed with coronary catheterization. These facts highlight the imperfections of conventional coronary angiography in capturing the complexity of coronary pathophysiology in women. Lack of clinician awareness of these unique aspects of the pathophysiology of CHD in women could lead to missed opportunities for diagnosis and appropriate treatment.

Another important sex difference in CHD pathophysiology pertains to spontaneous coronary artery dissection (SCAD). Women comprise 90% of all patients with SCAD [32, 46]. Further, SCAD has different precipitating factors based on sex (most commonly emotional triggers in women and physical triggers in men) [46] and presents more aggressively and with worse prognosis when associated with pregnancy [47].

Symptoms of CHD

It is common to refer to women as having "atypical symptoms" for CHD, but this approach also tends to marginalize women's cardiovascular health. It is necessary to remember that the descriptions of "typical" or "classic" angina were made from studies that included only men. Once we acknowledge this fact, we can understand that there are two patterns of CHD symptoms: a male pattern (which is well described in the literature and what clinicians are classically trained to recognize) and a female pattern (which is less well described, but with growing understanding in the contemporary era). One common misconception is that women with CHD do not present with chest pain. While it is true that more women than men will present with epigastric or back pain, or isolated dyspnea [48], contemporary studies have shown us that the majority of women with acute coronary syndromes do present with chest pain and that the proportion of women presenting with chest pain is not different than men's (87% vs 90%, respectively) [49]. However, women are more likely than men to present with three or more additional symptoms (such as dyspnea, dizziness, and numbness, among others) [49], which may "dilute" the focus from the chest pain, making the diagnosis less obvious for the woman and for healthcare providers.

Diagnostic Testing for CHD

With regard to diagnostic testing, important sex differences also exist and need to be acknowledged. Treadmill exercise testing is less accurate in women than men [50], perhaps partially owing to the aforementioned sex differences in CHD pathophysiology. Further, single-photon emission computed tomography (SPECT) interpretation is different, based on sex [51]. Women often have smaller left ventricle chambers, which can lead to underrepresentation of defects and false-negative results; or false-positive results due to breast tissue attenuation artifact. Notably, diagnostic accuracy of stress testing is usually determined based on correlation with presence and severity of angiographic coronary artery disease, which, as mentioned above, is not the only cause of ischemic chest pain in women. Thus, novel imaging modalities are needed in order to improve CHD diagnostic accuracy in women. Based on this need, recent studies have promoted innovative stress testing techniques. For example, it has been shown that women are twice as likely as men to develop myocardial ischemia from a mental stress test [52], highlighting the fact that ischemic triggers for women can be different and would not necessarily be identified with conventional stress testing.

CHD Treatment

On the treatment front, women with CHD are less likely than men to receive thrombolytics [53], coronary angiography [54], and percutaneous [55–57] and surgical coronary revascularization [54, 55], despite similar indications. In addition, women with acute coronary syndromes are less likely to be prescribed or continue taking statins [58], although men and women benefit similarly from this therapy [59]. Furthermore, while the majority of the literature has focused on sex differences, recent evidence shows us that we should also pay attention to gender: among people with premature CHD, those who had a more feminine gender score were more likely to suffer a reinfarction than those with a more masculine gender score [27]. These findings were present independently of a person's biological sex. Authors speculated that such gender differences in prognosis could be attributed to the higher stress levels associated with a feminine gender role in today's society.

The aforementioned facts, although well disseminated among sex and gender experts, are not usually taught as part of graduate or postgraduate curricula, leading to significant gaps in clinical practice. By creating a dedicated Women's Heart Health Team, healthcare institutions can bring these well-established issues to the forefront, engage clinicians, develop the necessary education and policy strategies, and help eliminate sex and gender gaps in cardiovascular care and outcomes.

Sex and Gender Differences in Other Types of Cardiovascular Diseases: Expanding the Scope of a Heart Team Beyond the Coronaries

Although CHD prevention, diagnosis, and treatment constitute the majority of cardiovascular clinical practice in most institutions, it is important to acknowledge that sex and gender differences have also been described in other types of cardiovascular diseases. Understanding these differences will expand the scope of a Women's Heart Health Team and will be briefly summarized below.

Heart Failure

Among ambulatory patients with heart failure, mortality is higher in women than men [60]. Women are twice as likely as men to have heart failure with preserved ejection fraction [19], owing to sex differences in cardiac structure, function, and metabolism, vascular aging, and immune system biology [61]. In addition, peripartum cardiomyopathy, a potentially morbid condition [62], is unique to women.

Pulmonary Hypertension

Women are four times more likely than men to develop pulmonary arterial hypertension (PAH) [63], although men with this condition have worse prognosis [64]. Women's predisposition appears to be due to sex hormone signaling and synthesis in the pulmonary circulation [65].

Valvular Heart Disease

Among patients with aortic stenosis, women are more likely to develop concentric left ventricular remodeling, while men tend to develop concentric or eccentric left ventricular hypertrophy [66]. Aortic stenosis surgery in women can be more technically demanding, due to smaller annuli size, increased need for aortic enlargement, and complications related to cardiopulmonary bypass. Further, women tend to be older, frailer, and more symptomatic than men at the time of referral for surgical aortic valve replacement (SAVR) [67] and are more likely to have a stroke in the postoperative period [68]. Conversely, among people with aortic stenosis referred for transcatheter aortic valve replacement (TAVR), women experience more vascular complications, blood transfusions, serious procedural complications, and a greater incidence of stroke but have lower rates of post-procedural

aortic regurgitation [69] and better long-term outcomes than men [70, 71]. For aortic regurgitation, it must be noted that utilizing guideline-based, non-indexed left ventricular dimensions to guide surgical indication in women is futile, since such ventricular dimensions are almost never reached in women, who often undergo surgery only after developing severe symptoms [72]. Postoperatively, late mortality is higher in women, suggesting that surgical correction should be considered at an earlier stage in women [72] and that left ventricular dimensions indexed to body size should be used to guide surgical decisions in women. Among people with mitral valve prolapse, women are less likely to have posterior leaflet prolapse or flail segments, but more likely to have leaflet thickening. In addition, for those with severe mitral regurgitation, women were less likely to receive mitral valve surgery [73], to have their valve repaired [74], and were more likely to have recurrence of significant regurgitation [75] and to die [73] when compared to men. Women appear to be referred for mitral valve surgery later in the disease process [75], and, as a result, mitral valve surgery restores normal life expectancy in men but not in women [76].

Arrhythmias

Women are more likely than men to have sick sinus syndrome, atrioventricular node reentrant tachycardia, and long QT-associated arrhythmias [77]. In atrial fibrillation, sex disparities also exist. Despite similar prevalence of disease between sexes, and the fact that symptom burden is greater [78, 79] and quality of life is worse [80] in women, women are less likely than men to be seen by a cardiologist or electrophysiologist or to receive catheter ablation and anticoagulation [81]. Among patients with heart failure with ejection fraction <35%, women are 16% less likely than men to be counseled for an implantable cardioverter-defibrillator for primary prevention of sudden cardiac death [82], although men and women benefit equally from the device [83]. In addition, in heart failure patients qualifying for cardiac resynchronization therapy (CRT), cardiac vein accessibility is higher in women, [84] and women derive greater benefit from the therapy than men [85]. Despite this, CRT utilization is greater in men than in women [86].

Diseases of the Aorta

Although thoracic aortic aneurysms (TAA) and abdominal aortic aneurysms (AAA) are more common in men, women with these conditions experience faster aneurysm growth [21, 22] and worse outcomes [21]. For example, for AAA, rupture rates are fourfold higher and occur at smaller aneurysm sizes in women than

men [87]. Further, women are less likely to be referred for elective, ruptured, or endovascular AAA repair than men [88–90], and once operated on, have a higher incidence of periprocedural complications [91]. For TAA, women experience a threefold increase in the risk of aneurysm dissection or rupture and 40% increase in mortality [92, 93].

Knowledge of these sex-based differences in cardiovascular diseases is the first step toward addressing institutional gaps and barriers in women's cardiovascular health, fueling the need for a dedicated Women's Heart Health Team to systematically address these issues. By doing so, the Heart Team has the potential to change institutional culture, engage staff, implement new programs and protocols, and motivate sex-based research to fill remaining knowledge gaps.

The University of Ottawa Heart Institute's Women's Heart Health Team

Understanding the necessity to emphasize the needs and unique aspects of cardiovascular disease in women in order to improve their health, the University of Ottawa Heart Institute (UOHI) launched the Canadian Women's Heart Health Centre in 2014 and the Women's Heart Health Team in 2016. The Centre and the Team are separate entities with different memberships but work synergistically toward improving the cardiovascular health of women.

The UOHI Women's Heart Health Team comprises cardiologists, anesthesiologists, cardiac surgeons, nurses, psychologists, exercise physiologists, managers, trainees, and women with lived experience in cardiovascular disease. Several of the team's healthcare professionals are clinician-scientists. The diverse membership ensures that all possible determinants of women's cardiovascular health are addressed and creates an environment that fosters creativity, innovation, and opportunity to create new approaches that cross traditional clinical silos. The deliverables observed in the first 2 years (at the time of writing of this chapter) since inception of the UOHI Women's Heart Health Team are summarized in Table 7.1. The achievements illustrated in Table 7.1 demonstrate the transformative effect of prioritization of women's health at the institutional level.

Barriers to a Women's Heart Health Team

A major barrier to initiating a Women's Heart Health Team is overcoming institutional culture, as any changes to current practice will require "buy-in" and prioritization from leadership and from staff. Furthermore, because the topic of "Women's Heart Health" is broad, determining priorities for action can be a time-consuming exercise and will depend on the strengths, weaknesses, and gaps observed in each

Table 7.1 Achievements of the University of Ottawa Heart Institute (UOHI)'s Women's Heart Health Team within 2 years of inception

Area	Achievements
Clinical care	Creation and incorporation of women-specific information about cardiovascular disease in inpatient discharge classes
	Establishment of the Women@Heart program, a community-based peer-support program for women with heart disease delivered by women with heart disease (peer leaders)[a]
	Development of the Inpatient Women@Heart, where women hospitalized at the UOHI receive a bedside visit by a peer leader, who provides support and advice[a]
	Establishment of the IMPROVE Postpartum Program, a health coaching program aimed at improving the cardiovascular health of women with recent diagnoses of hypertensive disorders of pregnancy or gestational diabetes[a]
	Establishing of the Champlain region's first Women's Heart Health Clinic, providing state-of-the-art care to women with or at risk for heart disease
Education	Co-hosting of the biennial Canadian Women's Heart Health Summit, Canada's first conference dedicated exclusively to the unique aspects of cardiovascular health and disease in women[a]
	Several lectures on various topics related to women's cardiovascular health delivered to trainees, staff physicians, and nurses
	Establishment of a Women's Heart Health Lecture Series as part of weekly Grand Rounds, in order to educate our healthcare providers and trainees about specific topics in women's cardiovascular health and improve the care delivered to women in our hospital. Then add another line to this row, saying: Establishment of a National Alliance for Knowledge Translation in Women's Heart Health, with the primary goal of developing innovative solutions to eliminate knowledge and practice gaps pertaining to cardiovascular health and disease in women[a]
Research	Chair in Women's Heart Health[a]
	Establishment of an annual lecture on Women's Cardiovascular Health Research as part of Research Rounds, to inspire our Institution's researchers and trainees to incorporate sex- and gender-based analyses in their research
	Incorporation of sex- and gender-based research into the core of the revised institutional research strategic plan
	Creation and dissemination of a "Sex- and gender-based research toolkit" for UOHI investigators
	3.7-fold increase in the number of manuscripts by UOHI investigators focusing on women or on sex differences in cardiovascular diseases
	Increase in the number of grant proposals from our Institution including sex and/or gender in the analytic plan to 80% of all submitted grants
Advocacy	Several lectures on women's heart health delivered to the community
	Creation of the "Women's heart health advocacy toolkit" for individuals who wish to advocate for women's heart health in their communities[a]

UOHI, University of Ottawa Heart Institute
[a]Indicates activities developed by the Canadian Women's Heart Health Centre

healthcare institution. There is also a lack of financial reimbursement and lack of "real-world" data to demonstrate a clinical advantage of this strategy. Many of these obstacles can be overcome with strong institutional support for multidisciplinary Women's Heart Health Teams, and ongoing research/quality improvement initiatives to document the successes of the Team's projects.

Conclusions

There are several sex- and gender-based disparities in cardiovascular diseases, although knowledge of such disparities is not uniformly translated to healthcare providers, leading to gaps in cardiovascular care and outcomes for women. Based on our experience at the University of Ottawa Heart Institute, creation of a dedicated multidisciplinary Women's Heart Health Team as part of strategic institutional prioritization of women's cardiovascular health has significant potential to change local culture, engage providers, enhance advocacy efforts, foster scientific inquiry, and improve clinical care for women. Institutions must evaluate their own strengths, weaknesses, and practice patterns in order to identify the most relevant needs, the necessary membership, and the strategy that will inform their Women's Heart Health Team. By bringing women's cardiovascular needs to the forefront, healthcare institutions can have a significant positive impact on the health and quality of life of women, helping dispel existing sex- and gender-based disparities in care. Further, Women's Heart Health Teams can help in the creation of niches and leadership opportunities for their staff/providers.

References

1. Teo KK, Cohen E, Buller C, Hassan A, Carere R, Cox JL, et al. Canadian Cardiovascular Society/Canadian Association of Interventional Cardiology/Canadian Society of Cardiac Surgery position statement on revascularization—multivessel coronary artery disease. Can J Cardiol. 2014;30:1482–91.
2. Hillis LD, Smith PK, Anderson JL, Bittl JA, Bridges CR, Byrne JG, et al. 2011 ACCF/AHA guideline for coronary artery bypass graft surgery. A report of the American College of Cardiology Foundation/American Heart Association task force on practice guidelines. Developed in collaboration with the American Association for Thoracic Surgery, Society of Cardiovascular Anesthesiologists, and Society of Thoracic Surgeons. J Am Coll Cardiol. 2011;58:e123–210.
3. Fihn SD, Blankenship JC, Alexander KP, Bittl JA, Byrne JG, Fletcher BJ, et al. 2014 ACC/AHA/AATS/PCNA/SCAI/STS focused update of the guideline for the diagnosis and management of patients with stable ischemic heart disease: a report of the American College of Cardiology/American Heart Association task force on practice guidelines, and the American Association for Thoracic Surgery, Preventive Cardiovascular Nurses Association, Society for Cardiovascular Angiography and Interventions, and Society of Thoracic Surgeons. J Thorac Cardiovasc Surg. 2015;149:e5–23.
4. Luckraz H, Norell M, Buch M, James R, Cooper G. Structure and functioning of a multidisciplinary "Heart Team" for patients with coronary artery disease: rationale and recommendations from a joint BCS/BCIS/SCTS working group. Eur J Cardiothorac Surg. 2015;48:524–9.
5. Webb J, Rodes-Cabau J, Fremes S, Pibarot P, Ruel M, Ibrahim R, et al. Transcatheter aortic valve implantation: a Canadian Cardiovascular Society position statement. Can J Cardiol. 2012;28:520–8.
6. Taylor C, Munro AJ, Glynne-Jones R, Griffith C, Trevatt P, Richards M, et al. Multidisciplinary team working in cancer: what is the evidence? BMJ. 2010;340:c951.
7. Freeman JV, Wang Y, Akar J, Desai N, Krumholz H. National trends in atrial fibrillation hospitalization, readmission, and mortality for medicare beneficiaries, 1999-2013. Circulation. 2017;135:1227–39.

8. Kesson EM, Allardice GM, George WD, Burns HJ, Morrison DS. Effects of multidisciplinary team working on breast cancer survival: retrospective, comparative, interventional cohort study of 13 722 women. BMJ. 2012;344:e2718.
9. Heart and Stroke Foundation of Canada. Ms. Understood. Heart & Stroke 2018 heart report. Available at: https://www.heartandstroke.ca/-/media/pdf-files/canada/2018-heart-month/hs_2018-heart-report_en.ashx.
10. McDonnell LA, Pipe AL, Westcott C, Perron S, Younger-Lewis D, Elias N, et al. Perceived vs actual knowledge and risk of heart disease in women: findings from a Canadian survey on heart health awareness, attitudes, and lifestyle. Can J Cardiol. 2014;30:827–34.
11. McDonnell LA, Turek M, Coutinho T, Nerenberg K, de Margerie M, Perron S, et al. Women's heart health: knowledge, beliefs, and practices of Canadian physicians. J Womens Health (Larchmt). 2018;27:72–82.
12. Barsheshet A, Brenyo A, Goldenberg I, Moss AJ. Sex-related differences in patients' responses to heart failure therapy. Nat Rev Cardiol. 2012;9:234–42.
13. Fazal L, Azibani F, Vodovar N, Cohen Solal A, Delcayre C, Samuel JL. Effects of biological sex on the pathophysiology of the heart. Br J Pharmacol. 2014;171:555–66.
14. Hoppe BL, Hermann DD. Sex differences in the causes and natural history of heart failure. Curr Heart Rep. 2003;5:193–9.
15. Bucholz EM, Butala NM, Rathore SS, Dreyer RP, Lansky AJ, Krumholz HM. Sex differences in long-term mortality after myocardial infarction: a systematic review. Circulation. 2014;130:757–67.
16. Dunlay SM, Roger VL. Gender differences in the pathophysiology, clinical presentation, and outcomes of ischemic heart failure. Curr Heart Fail Rep. 2012;9:267–76.
17. Rosen SE, Henry S, Bond R, Pearte C, Mieres JH. Sex-specific disparities in risk factors for coronary heart disease. Curr Atheroscler Rep. 2015;17:49.
18. Herz ND, Engeda J, Zusterzeel R, Sanders WE, O'Callaghan KM, Strauss DG, et al. Sex differences in device therapy for heart failure: utilization, outcomes, and adverse events. J Womens Health (Larchmt). 2015;24:261–71.
19. Scantlebury DC, Borlaug BA. Why are women more likely than men to develop heart failure with preserved ejection fraction? Curr Opin Cardiol. 2011;26:562–8.
20. Sanghavi M, Gulati M. Sex differences in the pathophysiology, treatment, and outcomes in IHD. Curr Atheroscler Rep. 2015;17:511.
21. Boczar K, Coutinho T. Sex considerations in aneurysm formation, progression and outcomes. Can J Cardiol. 2018;34(4):362–70.
22. Cheung K, Boodhwani M, Chan KL, Beauchesne L, Dick A, Coutinho T. Thoracic aortic aneurysm growth: role of sex and aneurysm etiology. J Am Heart Assoc. 2017;6(2):pii: e003792.
23. Coutinho T. Arterial stiffness and its clinical implications in women. Can J Cardiol. 2014;30:756–64.
24. Coutinho T, Borlaug BA, Pellikka PA, Turner ST, Kullo IJ. Sex differences in arterial stiffness and ventricular-arterial interactions. J Am Coll Cardiol. 2013;61:96–103.
25. Coutinho T, Pellikka PA, Bailey KR, Turner ST, Kullo IJ. Sex differences in the associations of hemodynamic load with left ventricular hypertrophy and concentric remodeling. Am J Hypertens. 2016;29:73–80.
26. Coutinho T, Yam Y, Chow BJW, Dwivedi G, Inacio J. Sex differences in associations of arterial compliance with coronary artery plaque and calcification burden. J Am Heart Assoc. 2017;6(8):pii: e006079.
27. Pelletier R, Khan NA, Cox J, Daskalopoulou SS, Eisenberg MJ, Bacon SL, et al. Sex versus gender-related characteristics: which predicts outcome after acute coronary syndrome in the young? J Am Coll Cardiol. 2016;67:127–35.
28. Reeves MJ, Bushnell CD, Howard G, Gargano JW, Duncan PW, Lynch G, et al. Sex differences in stroke: epidemiology, clinical presentation, medical care, and outcomes. Lancet Neurol. 2008;7:915–26.
29. Coutinho T, Lamai O, Nerenberg K. Hypertensive disorders of pregnancy and cardiovascular diseases: current knowledge and future directions. Curr Treat Options Cardiovasc Med. 2018;20:56.

30. Hilfiker-Kleiner D, Haghikia A, Nonhoff J, Bauersachs J. Peripartum cardiomyopathy: current management and future perspectives. Eur Heart J. 2015;36:1090–7.
31. Borlaug BA, Redfield MM. Diastolic and systolic heart failure are distinct phenotypes within the heart failure spectrum. Circulation. 2011;123:2006–13.
32. Saw J, Mancini GBJ, Humphries KH. Contemporary review on spontaneous coronary artery dissection. J Am Coll Cardiol. 2016;68:297–312.
33. Martins D, Nelson K, Pan D, Tareen N, Norris K. The effect of gender on age-related blood pressure changes and the prevalence of isolated systolic hypertension among older adults: data from NHANES III. J Gend Specif Med. 2001;4:10–3, 20.
34. Wenger N. Tailoring cardiovascular risk assessment and prevention for women: one size does not fit all. Glob Cardiol Sci Pract. 2017;2017:e201701.
35. Anand SS, Islam S, Rosengren A, Franzosi MG, Steyn K, Yusufali AH, et al. Risk factors for myocardial infarction in women and men: insights from the INTERHEART study. Eur Heart J. 2008;29:932–40.
36. Park TH, Ko Y, Lee SJ, Lee KB, Lee J, Han MK, et al. Identifying target risk factors using population attributable risks of ischemic stroke by age and sex. J Stroke. 2015;17:302–11.
37. He J, Ogden LG, Bazzano LA, Vupputuri S, Loria C, Whelton PK. Risk factors for congestive heart failure in US men and women: NHANES I epidemiologic follow-up study. Arch Intern Med. 2001;161:996–1002.
38. Palatini P, Mos L, Santonastaso M, Saladini F, Benetti E, Mormino P, et al. Premenopausal women have increased risk of hypertensive target organ damage compared with men of similar age. J Womens Health (Larchmt). 2011;20:1175–81.
39. Cheng S, Claggett B, Correia AW, Shah AM, Gupta DK, Skali H, et al. Temporal trends in the population attributable risk for cardiovascular disease: the atherosclerosis risk in communities study. Circulation. 2014;130:820–8.
40. Huxley R, Barzi F, Woodward M. Excess risk of fatal coronary heart disease associated with diabetes in men and women: meta-analysis of 37 prospective cohort studies. BMJ. 2006;332:73–8.
41. Huxley RR, Woodward M. Cigarette smoking as a risk factor for coronary heart disease in women compared with men: a systematic review and meta-analysis of prospective cohort studies. Lancet. 2011;378:1297–305.
42. Kurmann RD, Mankad R. Atherosclerotic heart disease in women with autoimmune rheumatologic inflammatory conditions. Can J Cardiol. 2018;34:381–9.
43. Reynolds HR, Srichai MB, Iqbal SN, Slater JN, Mancini GB, Feit F, et al. Mechanisms of myocardial infarction in women without angiographically obstructive coronary artery disease. Circulation. 2011;124:1414–25.
44. Pepine CJ, Ferdinand KC, Shaw LJ, Light-McGroary KA, Shah RU, Gulati M, et al. Emergence of nonobstructive coronary artery disease: a woman's problem and need for change in definition on angiography. J Am Coll Cardiol. 2015;66:1918–33.
45. Safdar B, D'Onofrio G, Dziura J, Russell RR, Johnson C, Sinusas AJ. Prevalence and characteristics of coronary microvascular dysfunction among chest pain patients in the emergency department. Eur Heart J Acute Cardiovasc Care. 2018:2048872618764418.
46. Tweet MS, Hayes SN, Pitta SR, Simari RD, Lerman A, Lennon RJ, et al. Clinical features, management, and prognosis of spontaneous coronary artery dissection. Circulation. 2012;126:579–88.
47. Tweet MS, Hayes SN, Codsi E, Gulati R, Rose CH, Best PJM. Spontaneous coronary artery dissection associated with pregnancy. J Am Coll Cardiol. 2017;70:426–35.
48. Canto JG, Goldberg RJ, Hand MM, Bonow RO, Sopko G, Pepine CJ, et al. Symptom presentation of women with acute coronary syndromes: myth vs reality. Arch Intern Med. 2007;167:2405–13.
49. Lichtman JH, Leifheit EC, Safdar B, Bao H, Krumholz HM, Lorenze NP, et al. Sex differences in the presentation and perception of symptoms among young patients with myocardial infarction: evidence from the VIRGO study (variation in recovery: role of gender on outcomes of young AMI patients). Circulation. 2018;137:781–90.

50. Kwok Y, Kim C, Grady D, Segal M, Redberg R. Meta-analysis of exercise testing to detect coronary artery disease in women. Am J Cardiol. 1999;83:660–6.
51. Garuba HA, Erthal F, Stadnick E, Alzahrani A, Chow B, deKemp R, et al. Optimizing risk stratification and noninvasive diagnosis of ischemic heart disease in women. Can J Cardiol. 2018;34:400–12.
52. Vaccarino V, Sullivan S, Hammadah M, Wilmot K, Al Mheid I, Ramadan R, et al. Mental stress-induced-myocardial ischemia in young patients with recent myocardial infarction: sex differences and mechanisms. Circulation. 2018;137:794–805.
53. Clarke KW, Gray D, Keating NA, Hampton JR. Do women with acute myocardial infarction receive the same treatment as men? BMJ. 1994;309:563–6.
54. Steingart RM, Packer M, Hamm P, Coglianese ME, Gersh B, Geltman EM, et al. Sex differences in the management of coronary artery disease. Survival and ventricular enlargement investigators. N Engl J Med. 1991;325:226–30.
55. Graham G, Xiao YY, Rappoport D, Siddiqi S. Population-level differences in revascularization treatment and outcomes among various United States subpopulations. World J Cardiol. 2016;8:24–40.
56. Khera S, Kolte D, Gupta T, Subramanian KS, Khanna N, Aronow WS, et al. Temporal trends and sex differences in revascularization and outcomes of ST-segment elevation myocardial infarction in younger adults in the United States. J Am Coll Cardiol. 2015;66:1961–72.
57. Pilgrim T, Heg D, Tal K, Erne P, Radovanovic D, Windecker S, et al. Age- and gender-related disparities in primary percutaneous coronary interventions for acute ST-segment elevation myocardial infarction. PLoS One. 2015;10:e0137047.
58. Carey IM, DeWilde S, Shah SM, Harris T, Whincup PH, Cook DG. Statin use after first myocardial infarction in UK men and women from 1997 to 2006: who started and who continued treatment? Nutr Metab Cardiovasc Dis. 2012;22:400–8.
59. Truong QA, Murphy SA, McCabe CH, Armani A, Cannon CP, Group TS. Benefit of intensive statin therapy in women: results from PROVE IT-TIMI 22. Circ Cardiovasc Qual Outcomes. 2011;4:328–36.
60. Sun LY, Tu JV, Coutinho T, Turek M, Rubens FD, McDonnell L, et al. Sex differences in outcomes of heart failure in an ambulatory, population-based cohort from 2009 to 2013. CMAJ. 2018;190:E848–54.
61. Beale AL, Meyer P, Marwick TH, Lam CSP, Kaye DM. Sex differences in cardiovascular pathophysiology: why women are overrepresented in heart failure with preserved ejection fraction. Circulation. 2018;138:198–205.
62. Azibani F, Sliwa K. Peripartum cardiomyopathy: an update. Curr Heart Fail Rep. 2018;15:297–306.
63. Mair KM, Johansen AK, Wright AF, Wallace E, MacLean MR. Pulmonary arterial hypertension: basis of sex differences in incidence and treatment response. Br J Pharmacol. 2014;171:567–79.
64. Benza RL, Miller DP, Gomberg-Maitland M, Frantz RP, Foreman AJ, Coffey CS, et al. Predicting survival in pulmonary arterial hypertension: insights from the registry to evaluate early and long-term pulmonary arterial hypertension disease management (REVEAL). Circulation. 2010;122:164–72.
65. Martin YN, Pabelick CM. Sex differences in the pulmonary circulation: implications for pulmonary hypertension. Am J Phys. 2014;306:H1253–64.
66. Treibel TA, Kozor R, Fontana M, Torlasco C, Reant P, Badiani S, et al. Sex dimorphism in the myocardial response to aortic stenosis. JACC Cardiovasc Imaging. 2018;11:962–73.
67. Dobson LE, Fairbairn TA, Plein S, Greenwood JP. Sex differences in aortic stenosis and outcome following surgical and transcatheter aortic valve replacement. J Womens Health (Larchmt). 2015;24:986–95.
68. Duncan AI, Lin J, Koch CG, Gillinov AM, Xu M, Starr NJ. The impact of gender on in-hospital mortality and morbidity after isolated aortic valve replacement. Anesth Analg. 2006;103:800–8.

69. Ferrante G, Pagnotta P, Petronio AS, Bedogni F, Brambilla N, Fiorina C, et al. Sex differences in postprocedural aortic regurgitation and mid-term mortality after transcatheter aortic valve implantation. Catheter Cardiovasc Interv. 2014;84:264–71.
70. Hayashida K, Morice MC, Chevalier B, Hovasse T, Romano M, Garot P, et al. Sex-related differences in clinical presentation and outcome of transcatheter aortic valve implantation for severe aortic stenosis. J Am Coll Cardiol. 2012;59:566–71.
71. Mihos CG, Klassen SL, Yucel E. Sex-specific considerations in women with aortic stenosis and outcomes after transcatheter aortic valve replacement. Curr Treat Options Cardiovasc Med. 2018;20:52.
72. Klodas E, Enriquez-Sarano M, Tajik AJ, Mullany CJ, Bailey KR, Seward JB. Surgery for aortic regurgitation in women. Contrasting indications and outcomes compared with men. Circulation. 1996;94:2472–8.
73. Avierinos JF, Inamo J, Grigioni F, Gersh B, Shub C, Enriquez-Sarano M. Sex differences in morphology and outcomes of mitral valve prolapse. Ann Intern Med. 2008;149:787–95.
74. Mokhles MM, Siregar S, Versteegh MI, Noyez L, van Putte B, Vonk AB, et al. Male-female differences and survival in patients undergoing isolated mitral valve surgery: a nationwide cohort study in the Netherlands. Eur J Cardiothorac Surg. 2016;50:482–7.
75. Chan V, Chen L, Elmistekawy E, Ruel M, Mesana TG. Determinants of late outcomes in women undergoing mitral repair of myxomatous degeneration. Interact Cardiovasc Thorac Surg. 2016;23:779–83.
76. Vassileva CM, McNeely C, Mishkel G, Boley T, Markwell S, Hazelrigg S. Gender differences in long-term survival of Medicare beneficiaries undergoing mitral valve operations. Ann Thorac Surg. 2013;96:1367–73.
77. Tadros R, Ton AT, Fiset C, Nattel S. Sex differences in cardiac electrophysiology and clinical arrhythmias: epidemiology, therapeutics, and mechanisms. Can J Cardiol. 2014;30:783–92.
78. Xiong Q, Proietti M, Senoo K, Lip GY. Asymptomatic versus symptomatic atrial fibrillation: a systematic review of age/gender differences and cardiovascular outcomes. Int J Cardiol. 2015;191:172–7.
79. Lip GY, Laroche C, Boriani G, Cimaglia P, Dan GA, Santini M, et al. Sex-related differences in presentation, treatment, and outcome of patients with atrial fibrillation in Europe: a report from the Euro Observational Research Programme Pilot survey on atrial fibrillation. Europace. 2015;17:24–31.
80. Jeong HK, Cho JG, Lee KH, Park HW, Kim MR, Lee KJ, et al. Determinants of quality of life in patients with atrial fibrillation. Int J Cardiol. 2014;172:e300–2.
81. Bhave PD, Lu X, Girotra S, Kamel H, Vaughan Sarrazin MS. Race- and sex-related differences in care for patients newly diagnosed with atrial fibrillation. Heart Rhythm. 2015;12:1406–12.
82. Hess PL, Hernandez AF, Bhatt DL, Hellkamp AS, Yancy CW, Schwamm LH, et al. Sex and race/ethnicity differences in implantable cardioverter-defibrillator counseling and use among patients hospitalized with heart failure: findings from the Get With The Guidelines-Heart Failure Program. Circulation. 2016;134:517–26.
83. Wilcox JE, Fonarow GC, Zhang Y, Albert NM, Curtis AB, Gheorghiade M, et al. Clinical effectiveness of cardiac resynchronization and implantable cardioverter-defibrillator therapy in men and women with heart failure: findings from IMPROVE HF. Circ Heart Fail. 2014;7:146–53.
84. Uhm JS, Park JW, Lee H, Kim TH, Youn JC, Joung B, et al. Cardiac vein accessibility according to heart diseases and sex: implications for cardiac resynchronization therapy. Pacing Clin Electrophysiol. 2016;39:513–21.
85. Zusterzeel R, Selzman KA, Sanders WE, O'Callaghan KM, Caños DA, Vernooy K, et al. Toward sex-specific guidelines for cardiac resynchronization therapy? J Cardiovasc Transl Res. 2016;9:12–22.
86. Sribhen K, Phankingthongkum R, Wannasilp N. Skeletal muscle disease as noncardiac cause of cardiac troponin T elevation. J Am Coll Cardiol. 2012;59:1334–5.
87. Sweeting MJ, Thompson SG, Brown LC, Powell JT, RESCAN Collaborators. Meta-analysis of individual patient data to examine factors affecting growth and rupture of small abdominal aortic aneurysms. Br J Surg. 2012;99:655–65.

88. Cowan JA Jr, Dimick JB, Henke PK, Rectenwald J, Stanley JC, Upchurch GR Jr. Epidemiology of aortic aneurysm repair in the United States from 1993 to 2003. Ann N Y Acad Sci. 2006;1085:1–10.
89. Katz DJ, Stanley JC, Zelenock GB. Gender differences in abdominal aortic aneurysm prevalence, treatment, and outcome. J Vasc Surg. 1997;25:561–8.
90. Dillavou ED, Muluk SC, Makaroun MS. A decade of change in abdominal aortic aneurysm repair in the United States: have we improved outcomes equally between men and women? J Vasc Surg. 2006;43:230–8.
91. Wisniowski B, Barnes M, Jenkins J, Boyne N, Kruger A, Walker PJ. Predictors of outcome after elective endovascular abdominal aortic aneurysm repair and external validation of a risk prediction model. J Vasc Surg. 2011;54:644–53.
92. Nienaber CA, Fattori R, Mehta RH, Richartz BM, Evangelista A, Petzsch M, et al. Gender-related differences in acute aortic dissection. Circulation. 2004;109:3014–21.
93. Davies RR, Goldstein LJ, Coady MA, Tittle SL, Rizzo JA, Kopf GS, et al. Yearly rupture or dissection rates for thoracic aortic aneurysms: simple prediction based on size. Ann Thorac Surg. 2002;73:17–27.

Heart Teams for Cardiac Imaging: The Right Test at the Right Time for the Right Patient

8

Daniel Juneau, Benjamin J. W. Chow, Rob Beanlands, and Andrew Michael Crean

Introduction

Since the discovery of X-rays in 1895 by Wilhelm Röntgen, medical imaging has not only grown tremendously in the diagnostic possibilities it offers but also in the complexity and challenges it presents. Imaging now plays a key role in all medical specialties. Cardiology is no exception. Advances in computed tomography (CT), magnetic resonance imaging (MRI), ultrasound (US), single-photon emission tomography (SPECT), and positron emission tomography (PET) have led us to a better understanding of cardiac function, structure, and physiopathology, as well as enabling decision-making for patient management.

For some time now, modern medical imaging has evolved past the point where a single person can pretend to be an expert in the field as a whole. The practice of medical imaging is now split between dedicated medical imaging specialists (radiologist and nuclear medicine/molecular imaging physician) who dedicate their whole career to the imaging field, and clinicians with advanced training in more well-defined sub-fields (such as a cardiologist with advanced training in one or more cardiac imaging modalities). The practice of medicine itself is also evolving;

D. Juneau
Centre Hospitalier de l'Université de Montréal (CHUM), Department of Nuclear Medicine, Montreal, QC, Canada

Division of Cardiology, University of Ottawa Heart Institute, Ottawa, ON, Canada
e-mail: daniel.juneau@umontreal.ca

B. J. W. Chow · R. Beanlands · A. M. Crean (✉)
Division of Cardiology, University of Ottawa Heart Institute, Ottawa, ON, Canada
e-mail: acrean@ottawaheart.ca

© Springer Nature Switzerland AG 2019
T. Mesana (ed.), *Heart Teams for Treatment of Cardiovascular Disease*,
https://doi.org/10.1007/978-3-030-19124-5_8

patients are living longer, and conditions that used to be acute or untreatable are becoming chronic. This has led to the emergence of more complex cases, which in turn require a greater integration of a more diverse team of specialists working together to achieve the best outcome for the patient.

The imaging world might already be a step ahead when it comes to the concept of the heart team and multidisciplinary work; after all, medical imaging has always been teamwork. With a few exceptions, medical imaging usually involves two different healthcare professionals: a clinician, or referring physician, and a medical imaging specialist, or consultant. They both have roles, and only together can they provide the best care for the patient. First, the clinician must define and provide a clear question to the imaging specialist. What are we trying to learn? What is the aim of this test? How will the results be used? He or she must also provide background information on the anatomy and physiology of the particular patient under investigation. In turn, the imaging specialist must use this information to the fullest to select the right test, the right imaging protocol, and to provide the best possible report/interpretation. Lastly, the clinician will need to put the results into clinical context and use it to guide therapy and decision-making. This may well be the most challenging portion of the process, and only when both clinicians and imaging specialists work in a fully integrated manner can the maximum benefit be derived for the patient.

In this chapter, we explore how the heart team concept can be used to its fullest in cardiac imaging and how it can help us obtain the maximal benefit for patient care: *the right test for the right patient.* We will cover several major aspects of cardiac imaging, from patient selection to study interpretation. Two different paradigms of the heart team in cardiac imaging will be discussed. The first will be the "imaging heart team," a specialized team dedicated to cardiac imaging, which includes members with specialized training in all cardiac imaging modalities and all aspect of cardiac imaging (test selection, imaging protocol, study interpretation, quality control/assurance, etc.). The second will look into the integration of cardiac imaging specialist(s) in other heart teams. This second approach is a logical step in a medical world growing ever more reliant on advanced imaging. One of the first changes toward that integration will be the switch from the medical imaging specialist as a consultant to the medical imaging specialist as a full member of the heart team. This is an important change in perception and mentality that both imaging specialists and clinicians must embrace to derive the greatest benefit from the heart team concept.

Patient Selection

The role of the heart team in cardiac imaging starts well before the actual imaging procedure with the most fundamental concern, patient selection. Appropriateness criteria issued by the specialist societies provide a framework governing optimal test selection. However, guidelines are not tablets of stone. Local circumstances and clinical judgment must always inform the choice of imaging procedure. A team approach to patient selection is likely to result not only in a more optimized

approach for the patient but also in a better use of local resources. While the imaging specialist may have the most knowledge of the tests themselves and their relative strengths and weaknesses, the clinician has the most knowledge about the patients themselves. Working together ensures that the heart team correctly identifies the patients who will benefit from cardiac imaging and those who will benefit from more advanced testing. The first and most important question is: what does the clinician want to know? This basic information—while it may seem obvious to the referring physician—may not always be so clear to the medical imaging specialist. Many imaging requisitions provide little or no useful clinical information, and despite literature confirming a significant impact on image interpretation [1, 2], the problem remains [3, 4]. In addition to providing the necessary background (symptoms, pertinent history, and prior testing), the clinician should always strive to convey his/her reasoning to the imaging specialist. Simply stating a patient has dyspnea or chest pain is rarely enough information to make an informed choice; these symptoms can be associated with a wide range of conditions. Defining a clear question and/or objective will ensure that the appropriate patient gets the appropriate imaging. What does the clinician need, and what can imaging provide? In occasional difficult cases, the question may be particularly nuanced, and it is important that this is transmitted to the imaging specialist if an equally nuanced report is desired. Working together as a heart team leads to many advantages in this regard; at a minimum, it facilitates the exchange and flow of information and leads to a better understanding of what is required/expected from all parties.

A heart team approach to patient selection will also make it easier to discuss the pertinence (or otherwise), of imaging in some patients. This discussion should take into account not only the resources available at each institution (such as the available modalities and protocols) but also the relative expertise and experience in the modality available locally. Reader experience has a significant impact on imaging interpretation, and published sensitivity/specificity figures from an experienced reference center may not always translate well to the local context [5]. This kind of information may not be known to the referring clinician but should be readily apparent to the heart imaging team. A team approach will also make it easier to establish which symptoms require investigation. Many organizations have tried to establish guidelines along these lines and to define scenarios where imaging should be restricted or reconsidered. These include initiative such as "Choosing Wisely" (http://www.choosingwisely.org/), "Image Wisely" (https://www.image-wisely.org/), and "Image Gently" (https://www.imagegently.org/), which all aim to promote appropriate practices and avoid unnecessary procedures, including medical imaging. Developing and applying these guidelines, however, requires a team approach, with input from both clinicians and imaging specialists, since generic rules and recommendations cannot be applied blindly to a specific patient. Generally, when acting only as a consultant, it is much simpler for the imaging specialist to simply perform whatever test was requested rather than to deny testing. This is particularly true when it is complicated, arduous, or simply time-consuming to track down the referring physician to discuss the pertinence of a given test in a given patient. In an acute or critical setting, when the imaging specialist does not

necessarily carry the full clinical responsibility for a patient, it is often much easier to simply perform the test as ordered, but not necessarily the right approach for the patient. This suboptimal testing generates additional costs for the health system and may expose the patient to unnecessary stress, radiation, and risks of complications/side effects. "Acquiescent imaging" of this kind is, unfortunately, not unusual in fee-for-service environments and represents an abdication on the part of the imager to fulfill the roles of "Experts" and "Health Advocates" (such roles are mandated in some jurisdictions by professional societies such as the Royal College of Physicians and Surgeons in Canada).

The heart team makes it much easier to come to a decision to forego unnecessary testing in a patient and also helps to ensure that the whole team is aligned in decision-making. This yields consistent rather than conflicting information for the patient regarding the necessity of testing (a situation which otherwise may have engendered doubts and eroded the trust between the patient and the medical team). While testing that is unlikely to have an impact on patient treatment and clinical decision-making should usually not be performed, some exceptions may occur. Patient (or even physician) reassurance may be a reasonable goal in some situations. Should we deny all testing to an asymptomatic 40-year-old man whose father died from a myocardial infarction in his 40s, if the stress and anxiety he feels is negatively impacting his quality of life? These considerations also need to be part of the discussion.

Beyond patient-specific care, the heart team can also help elaborate tools that help in patient and test selection. These can include computerized imaging requisition processes. In their most basic form, these systems simply duplicate the paper requisition electronically. However, it is also possible to implement decision-assistance algorithms in these systems, which help guide clinicians. These systems often include "hard stops," where, if insufficient information (or information that does not support the selected test) is provided, the system does not allow the imaging request to be routed to the imaging department. The focus of these systems needs to be on physician education however; otherwise, these "hard stops" can lead to misuse of the system by modifying information to get the desired test—bringing us back to the problem of insufficient/inadequate clinical information! When properly implemented, these systems are generally well accepted by clinicians and can lead to a decrease in inappropriate testing, an improvement in the quality/quantity of clinical information provided, and a decrease in inappropriate or low-yield testing [6–9].

Test Selection

The next logical step after patient selection is test selection. Having established that a given patient requires cardiac imaging, it becomes the role of the heart imaging team to determine which test would be most appropriate. Clinicians rarely think in terms of imaging modality when they see a patient. They usually focus on symptoms or specific disease entities and establish a differential diagnosis around which

they work. The imaging heart team can help in this aspect; they can be a proactive actor in test selection, helping the clinicians by organizing and presenting the available cardiac imaging tests and protocols in a way that clinicians are able to recognize and easily use.

At this stage, just as with patient selection, it is crucial for the heart imaging team to have a clear understanding of what the clinician wants to know, a clear question or request being the best start to appropriate test selection. Understanding what knowledge will be gained, how it will be used, and how it may (or may not) modify patient treatment will also help the imaging team make an informed decision. The cost-effectiveness and potential downstream resource utilization that comes with imaging also need to be considered. This is especially important for hospital administrators and provincial/third-party payers, with the implementation of performance-based reimbursement in many jurisdictions. This has led to an increase in interest and publications in cost-effectiveness analysis in the cardiac imaging field [10–13]. These studies and analyses, however, have limitations, often comparing only selected modalities. Their applicability may often be limited, since costs and access can vary widely from one jurisdiction to another. Lastly, these analyses—while valid at a population level—may not take into account patient-specific characteristics and conditions. Thus, it falls on the heart imaging team to incorporate all available data, including patient-specific data, in order to engage with the clinicians in a discussion that will lead to optimal test selection.

The imaging heart team also needs to take into account the accuracy and prognostic value of the different tests, again considering situation and patient-specific conditions, before selecting a test. This is especially true as we test individuals at both extremes of pre-test probability. Bayesian theory informs us that, at these extremes, a test with a very high positive or negative likelihood ratio will be required to have a significant impact on post-test probability, potentially justifying the use of more advanced (and often costlier) cardiac imaging tests [14].

Another important way in which the heart team can help achieve proper test selection is through the preparation and use of imaging guidelines. The involvement of the heart team begins with guideline development; input from all stakeholders is crucial to the elaboration of a document that will be useful. Several specialties and subspecialties need to be involved in order to address the complexity of modern medicine and imaging. Symptoms rarely fit into neat diagnostic compartments, and choosing to focus on a favored modality at the exclusion of the rest leads to disengagement of other specialists from the process that creates workable appropriateness criteria. Diagnostic "favouritism" of this sort may also lead to reduced use and acceptance of the recommendations. Having multiple guidelines, each one dealing in parallel with their modality or specific field, approaching the same situation in their own unique way, also leads to confusion for the clinicians who use the guidelines to guide practice.

The ideal approach is reflected in the recent appropriate use criteria (AUC) guidelines of the American College of Cardiology (ACC), which are multi-modality and involved expert stakeholders from multiple fields in their elaboration and review process [15–17]. The AUC methodology is central to constructing multi-modality

guidelines [18]. Putting these AUC guidelines into practice also favors a heart imaging team approach. There are often multiple appropriate tests/modalities in a single population, and the nuance and subtlety of each test cannot be accounted for in the AUC. Patient-related factors, ranging from physical characteristics (e.g. body habitus) to biological status (e.g. renal function, allergies), can have a crucial impact on patient and test selection. It is impossible for the AUC to cover the nearly limitless possibilities, hence the need for a refined ability to select the right patient, and the right test. Only by combining the expert knowledge of the imaging specialist and the clinician's intimate knowledge of the patient can optimal patient and test selection be achieved.

Imaging Protocols

Imaging protocols play integral roles in the imaging process, particularly so in cardiac imaging. Protocol development can greatly benefit from a heart team approach. Technology and protocols are evolving quickly, to a point where it has become difficult for a single person to be an expert in all available exams/protocols. A team approach should incorporate imaging specialists, technologists, and imaging physicists to ensure the optimal use of available resources and to assist in the design of optimized protocols. A well-scripted process enables the heart imaging team to fine-tune the imaging protocol to best answer the clinical query for any given patient in any given setting—instead of simply applying generic protocols to every situation: *the right test for the right patient in the right setting.* This is particularly true for cardiac imaging. For example, cardiac magnetic resonance (CMR) can be used to investigate multiple aspects of myocardial function and structure—or be used for tissue characterization—but can be quite time-consuming, with a full study running upward of 60 minutes. Not every sequence is useful in every clinical scenario, however, and through a heart team approach, it is possible to select the most appropriate sequences, making the examination more efficient, more cost-effective, and more patient-friendly. Similarly, when considering CT in a pregnant woman, a modified protocol can be designed, minimizing radiation exposure to the fetus and taking into account the hemodynamic changes associated with pregnancy that may alter the dynamics of contrast delivery. Shortened protocols can also be used in unstable patients; for example, using CT instead of MR or transesophageal echocardiography in an unstable and possibly dissecting patient. Sometimes an abbreviated protocol, while theoretically suboptimal, may still provide the core information needed to guide further management.

A team approach is implicit in the development of hybrid imaging platforms. Advances in hardware, including the introduction of PET/CT, SPECT/CT, and PET/MR, have opened up nearly endless possibilities for the simultaneous assessment of anatomical and functional data. With these possibilities come multiple questions: why do we need multiple modalities in this patient and what is the added value of this approach? Which modalities should we combine? How should this be

achieved—hybrid imaging, sequential imaging? The skills required for quality control and operation of one of the two fused image modalities may be quite different from that of the other. Future technologist and physician training will likely have to become more organ/system-focused rather than simply modality-based. Having different specialists working as an imaging heart team, to develop and optimize these protocols together, is the only way to ensure an optimal use of resources and a proper integration of all the information.

Many cardiac imaging procedures require stress testing (either exercise or pharmacological) and patient monitoring. A team approach will ensure the best protocols are selected for each patient, minimizing risks and delays. This can range from simple changes (using dobutamine instead of adenosine or dipyridamole in a patient with bronchospasm) to the much more complex. For example, in a young patient with suspected coronary spasm, SPECT myocardial perfusion imaging (MPI) might be performed, hoping to reproduce the symptoms and objectify ischemia. This would, of course, require exercise stress testing rather than pharmacological stress, and would mean that there might be further deviation from a standard exercise stress MPI, with tracer injection being performed upon achieving symptoms rather than 85% of the estimated maximum heart rate. This degree of customization is most easily achieved through the heart imaging team approach.

Physicists and technologists are also vital members of the imaging heart team, with important roles to play. Physicists have an integral role in the development of new protocols as well as troubleshooting technically challenging scans. Their integration into the imaging heart team is only logical. They also have an important part in the quality assurance and quality control of cardiac imaging. This is a critical aspect of all imaging procedures. Including physicists in the imaging heart team ensures they have a better understanding of how the machines and protocols are used. It also helps ensure that imaging physicians truly understand the importance of quality assurance/quality control procedures and the potential impact of not doing them properly or regularly.

Technologists also need to be fully integrated into the imaging heart team. They may well be the only ones to interact directly with a patient during the procedure. It is critical for them to understand what is being done and why—particularly when the heart team chooses to deviate from what would be considered "standard" testing. Patients will often ask technologists about the procedure, and these imaging staff need to be comfortable and confident in giving accurate replies. Being part of the imaging heart team helps to ensure that the technologists can provide their input when it comes to protocol design and implementation; then they can provide their own unique point of view. Being part of the heart team will also help to ensure that they have (and know that they have), the support of the physicians. Open communication lines between the technologists as part of the heart team minimize misunderstandings, delays, and incorrectly performed studies. This is important as day-to-day cardiac imaging often requires small, last-minute adjustments to imaging protocols for optimal image acquisition.

Working Together: A Historical Perspective on the Need for a Strong Partnership Between Clinicians and Imaging Specialists

The need for cardiac imaging teams cannot be appreciated without fully appreciating the historical evolution of cardiac imaging and, at times, the tense relationships between those who claim to be its greatest proponents [19, 20]. Both ultrasound and angiography were initially developed under the more general auspices of radiology, and 25 years ago it was not uncommon in some countries for both echocardiography and angiography (including coronary intervention) to be performed by radiologists. Indeed, one of the authors of this chapter performed his first 500 cardiac catheterizations under the supervision of a cardiac radiologist. However, it is a truism that those who drive innovation and research in an area are likely to become its leaders, and this was true for echocardiography and cardiac catheterization, which rapidly became the province of cardiology. The more recent emergence of cross-sectional cardiac imaging with CT and CMR, however, has seen a move by radiology to try to reclaim some of the ground that it has lost—and in many places unseemly battles have broken out between the two specialties for overall control, with skirmishes focusing on training [21, 22] and the potential for self-referral [23–25]. The only way to prevent this kind of internecine warfare is to form imaging teams to harness the undoubted strengths of both types of specialists. In places where this has happened, the benefits to both the patients and the fellows-in-training are obvious.

Study Interpretation and Reporting

Cardiology-radiology or cardiology-nuclear medicine team partnerships are likely to take slightly different forms depending upon local circumstances. At one end of the spectrum, radiology may act as the "safety net" for noncardiologic findings and will provide reads of the lungs, bones, and other non-cardiac structures for cardiac CT and MR performed (or whole-body imaging in the case of FDG PET). At the other end of the spectrum, cardiac imaging fellowship-trained radiologists will also read an agreed proportion of the studies for cardiac findings. The presence of PACS systems makes the "shared overread" of cases straightforward since the radiologist does not have to be present at the scanner or even in the same building to issue the noncardiac report. However, it is vital that the member of the team responsible for the *cardiac* portion of the exam is in the vicinity of the scanner, or at least immediately available, as many cases will require ad hoc decision-making and protocol optimization depending upon patient qualities such as cardiac rhythm and breath-holding capacity.

The advantage of a separate radiologic/nuclear medicine read for the the noncardiac findings is readily apparent (Fig. 8.1). Many years of training and exposure to noncardiac pathology result in a radiology opinion that is likely to be more accurate and nuanced than a cardiologic interpretation of the same noncardiac finding. Not

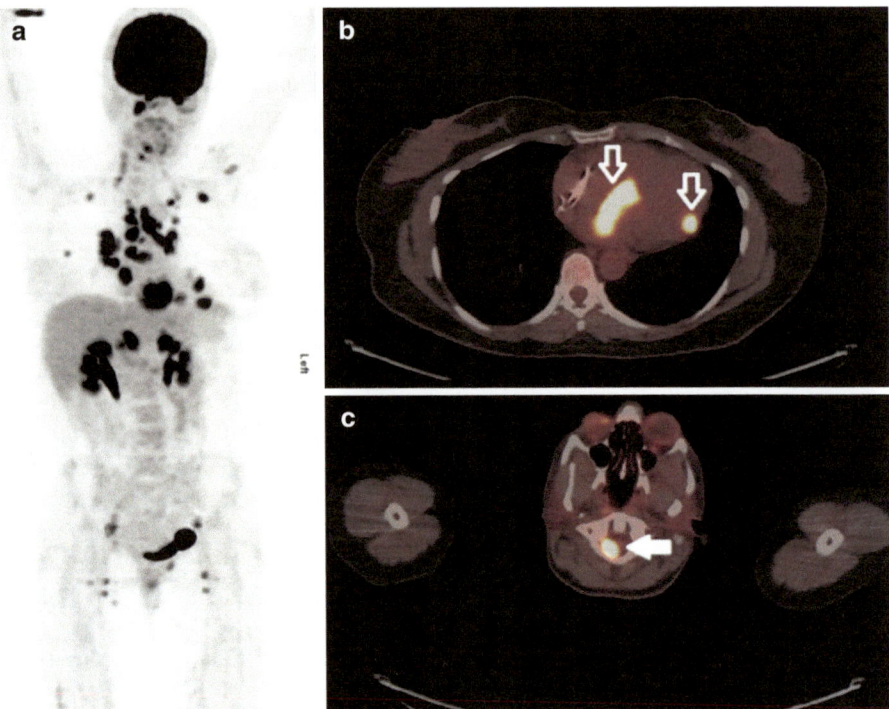

Fig. 8.1 (**a–c**) Positron emission tomography and computed tomography (PET-CT) with 18F-fluorodeoxyglucose (18F-FDG) images in a patient with previously diagnosed and treated cardiac sarcoidosis presenting with recurring cardiac symptoms. In addition to undergoing cardiac 18F-FDG PET-CT imaging, the patient also underwent whole-body imaging, which was reviewed by a nuclear medicine physician. Maximum intensity projection images (**a**) demonstrate multiple foci of uptake consistent with active cardiac and extra-cardiac sarcoidosis, with involvement of the lungs, nodes, and heart (**b**, white arrow contours). Whole-body imaging also revealed the presence of spinal cord involvement (**c**, white arrow), consistent with neurosarcoidosis, which is a rare but potentially serious complication of sarcoidosis. This crucial finding might have gone unreported if whole-body images had not been acquired or properly reviewed. The example illustrates the importance of imaging specialists with different talents working together as a team for the benefit of the patient. Case courtesy of Dr. David Birnie and the Cardiac Sarcoidosis Multi-Center Prospective Cohort Trial (CHASM-CS, NCT01477359)

only is this of obvious benefit to the patient, but it also represents an important educational opportunity for the cardiology fellows when they read out with radiology staff. This cross-fertilization of knowledge is by no means unidirectional, since radiology trainees equally benefit from the deep knowledge of cardiac pathology, physiology, and management that they are exposed to when reading with cardiology staff. Since the radiologic reader will inevitably look at the cardiac findings—even when only reporting the noncardiac portion—every study is effectively double-read, which stands as an excellent quality control measure.

Potential disadvantages of a split read can include a lack of cohesion between reports, or a staggered output of reports a few days apart. This might lead a referring

clinician to think she or he had already read a comprehensive report without realizing that a supplementary report for noncardiac findings was still outstanding (potentially with actionable findings). Some institutions solve this by aiming for same-day issuance of both the cardiac and the supplemental findings report, as well as by making clear reference to the presence of a supplementary report in the summary of the main cardiac report.

Ideal Reporting Environment

Modern imaging is by its very essence multi-modality. Many readers will have both primary and secondary areas of imaging expertise, one-day reading echo or nuclear, then perhaps CMR and CT. In order to maximize trainees' learning opportunities, it is advantageous to have a common reading area for all modalities so that truly comparative imaging may occur at any point in the day. This facilitates expert discussion for difficult cases *before* the report is issued, and trainees learn much about the relative strengths and weaknesses of various techniques in this way. It also models the concept of "honorable" professional uncertainty for trainees, in which asking a colleague for a second opinion becomes appreciated as a source of strength, not weakness.

Disadvantages of a common reading area include noise and temperature (many computers emitting heat) and both of these factors need to be considered in room design. One solution is a modular structure which allows the space to be opened or subdivided as required by numbers and for control of noise (for example, for teaching sessions). Overall, however, the strengths of the common reading area outweigh the disadvantages—and the ability to access multiple specialists by visiting a single area is greatly valued by in-hospital staff in need of an imaging consultation on their patients.

Communication of Results to Referrers, Colleagues, and Patients

Communication is key to the effectiveness of a heart imaging team. Regular operational meetings of the cardiac imaging team not only fosters a sense of communality, but is an opportunity to discuss protocols, review difficult cases, and conduct quality assurance. External communication from the team to the referring physician is no less important. As imaging teams grow in size there is a danger that reporting styles grow more disparate. Just as protocols are largely formalized, there is benefit to considering a common approach to reporting so that referring physicians quickly become accustomed to the report format and know where to look for the information that interests them the most. Many centers have moved away from the free-text reporting style (sometimes unkindly referred to as "stream of consciousness") that has been historically common amongst radiology reports. Many cardiovascular imagers prefer to use instead a structured template with predefined subject fields and subfields. Not only does this lend clarity and uniformity to reporting

style across the team members, but it also acts as a way to enter and code data into a back-end database which, being searchable, is invaluable for future research and quality control.

Modern cardiovascular medicine is complex, and management decisions are often predicated upon the results of imaging findings (Fig. 8.2). The standard for difficult decision-making is the multidisciplinary conference, and the heart imaging team should be central to this. The development of a team means that conferences do not need to be postponed by personal absence or vacation of a "key" reader. These conferences also act as a further form of quality control, since public presentation of study images not infrequently leads to a re-interpretation of their significance and provides a learning opportunity for the entire team. They are also a vital piece of team "advertising" and an opportunity to subtly (and occasionally not so subtly) remind surgical and interventional colleagues that imaging consultants are not simply passive medical photographers!

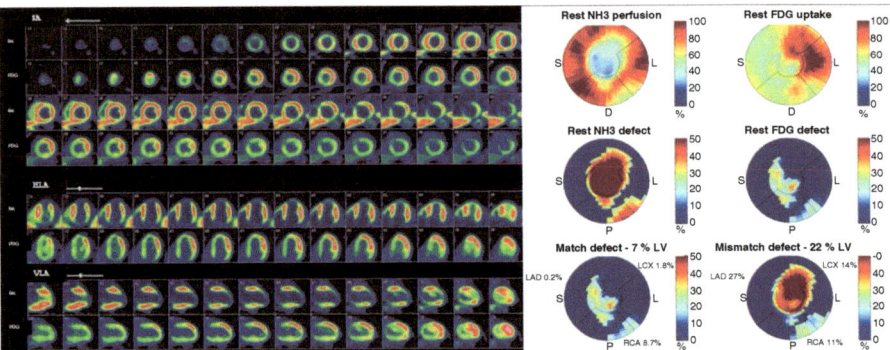

Fig. 8.2 Imaging to aid complex decision-making. Rest N^{13}-ammonia (Rst, top row) and F-18-fluorodeoxyglucose (FDG, bottom row) PET viability study in corresponding short axis (SA), horizontal long axis (HLA), and vertical long axis (VLA) slices, performed in a patient with documented multivessel disease and severe LV dysfunction to aid in revascularization decision-making. Perfusion images demonstrate moderate to severe reduction in tracer uptake in the mid to apical anterior and anterolateral walls, as well as the apex and apical inferior wall (LAD territory). There is also moderate reduction in uptake in the basal to mid inferolateral wall (RCA/LCx territory). The FDG images demonstrate FDG uptake in the mid to apical anterior wall and apex as well as in the basal to mid inferolateral wall. Polar maps of rest ammonia perfusion (top left) and corresponding rest ammonia defect (middle left), as well as rest F-18-FDG uptake (top right) and corresponding rest FDG defect (middle right) are provided. Our physicists, who created this software, incorporated a method of automatic calculation of the extent of mismatch between perfusion and viability. This is very helpful in reducing interobserver variability. The matched defect (bottom left) corresponds to a total scar score of 7% of LV myocardium, while the mismatch defect suggests that 22% of the ventricular myocardium is hibernating. Revascularization decisions are often difficult in patients with poor LV function as the immediate surgical risk is high. However, given the significant amount of hibernating myocardium, it was recommended that the patient proceed with coronary artery bypass grafting. Decision making for this patient was strengthened by teamwork involving imagers, physicists, and surgeons. (From Wiefels et al. [27]. Used with permission from Springer Nature)

Heart imaging team involvement in rounds is most developed in the areas of structural heart disease and adult congenital heart disease (ACHD), both high-risk areas of decision-making, and—in the case of ACHD—without large bodies of data to guide management. Surprisingly, there has been a relative under-involvement of the imaging team in other areas of cardiology including valvular heart disease, heart failure, and transplant. Furthermore, revascularization decisions are often made upon the basis of imaging study reports, but only rarely after conference has reviewed data presented by an imaging specialist. As such, there remain under-exploited opportunities for integration of the imaging team with other heart teams.

One area of communication which is readily overlooked is the issue of communicating findings with patients. In the past, an imager was often not directly involved in conveying test results to patients, but the era of patient access to the electronic medical record (EMR) has changed this irrevocably [26]. It now behooves an imager to be aware that the report may be read directly by the patient, even before it has been discussed with them by the ordering physician. Generally, this scenario is avoided by building into the EMR the requirement for the requesting physician to "release" the report to the patient, once reviewed. However, the authors wonder whether or not a non-technical summary appended to the end of the report (even if only a few lines) might be helpful to patient–physician relationships. If we can write patient information forms for research studies at the comprehension level of the general public, it should not prove too difficult (or time-consuming) to do the same for the reports we issue.

Training and Education

Traditionally, cardiac imagers have been trained in silos that were usually modality-based. Fellowship would consist of a year of echo, or a year of nuclear cardiology, or some other modality. There is no doubt that expertise can only be gained by volume and immersion, and yet this rigid educational format represents a lost opportunity to provide the next generation of imagers with the skills they are going to need. Expertise in every imaging modality is impractical to develop, as the time penalty is too great to achieve this in a single fellowship. More reasonable would be to ask trainees to declare one modality as a major interest and one as a minor interest. Twelve months of solid fellowship should provide adequate competency at those levels. Those who seek major competency in two modalities will perhaps have to accept that this requires a second year of fellowship for all but the most gifted. Two-year fellowships would thus grant major competency in two modalities and possibly minor competence in a third.

Perhaps this is also the right time to ask whether our model of training remains fit for purpose. Traditionally, fellowships have been very heavily service and research driven, and there is no doubt that the apprenticeship model has served us well. An apprenticeship model works particularly well for very high-volume services such as echo and nuclear, where the full spectrum of pathology can be encountered in a fairly compressed period of time. The model works less well for cardiac CT and

MRI, unless in a large center (>2000 cases per year for each), with a danger that fellowship graduates have not truly experienced all the complexities posed, both technical and clinicopathological. Although we would not advocate against the traditional service-based apprenticeship, perhaps there is something to be learned from the British Radiology Academies. Set up a few years ago in response to a dramatic shortage of trained radiologists, these bodies have collated vast amounts of teaching materials from content experts and centralized these resources in a way which enables access to any trainee anywhere in the country. Traditional geographic barriers to learning are surmounted, and the most instructive cases are available (with prepared commentary) to everyone. Why should a trainee in a smaller center have seen only one or two CMR cases of cardiac amyloidosis (for example) when a trainee in a larger center may have seen 20? A centralized and curated case repository is needed in many countries, particularly for cardiac CT, CMR, and PET.

As valuable as case collections would be to training, to stop there would be to miss the full potential of the Internet as a tool for instruction. Sites such as Coursera, Udemy, and Khan Academy are just a few that demonstrate the power and possibility of online instruction. One might imagine the potential of a "Cardiac Imaging Virtual University" where the very best teachers presented talks on topics with which they have the greatest expertise. Supplemented with recorded monthly real-time webinars, fellows-in-training could benefit from the accumulated knowledge of the country's most proficient imagers. A topic of difficulty could be watched and re-watched until fully understood. Real-time journal clubs or guest lectures could take place occasionally, bringing an entire country's imaging trainees together face-to-face. World experts from other countries could be invited to record talks to supplement existing lectures. Indeed, it would not be too fanciful to imagine that an entire curriculum for each imaging modality could be constructed and uniformly delivered to the trainees of the whole country as a supplement to their daily work schedule. The need for imaging educational champions to formalize a structure of this kind has never been greater. One hundred years from now, we shall look back at our current methods of training and frown in disbelief at how inefficient and geographically patchy they were.

Quality Control

Quality control is of fundamental importance in imaging. As modalities advance in both physical complexity and the complexity of image processing and reconstruction algorithms, there is an ever-present danger of data misrepresentation by the software to the readers. Fake data is as much a problem in imaging as fake news is on Facebook! Physics support is integral in preventing this from happening, particularly in nuclear cardiology and CMR. Cardiac PET is a good example of a fast-moving area requiring highly technical knowledge to assure that image data are acquired, processed, displayed, and interpreted in the correct manner. It is not unreasonable to suggest that physics team membership should be an auditable quality standard for all advanced imaging centers. The authors are lucky enough to

work at a center where physicists are front-and-center members of the heart imaging team; they are highly visible and easily accessible, attend daily clinical conferences alongside the imagers, give regular rounds on topics in imaging physics, and both drive their own and others' research programs forward to the general benefit of the whole team.

Research

Imaging research drives innovation and development within the specialty and is part of the core mission of the heart imaging team. Open and collegial working results in an atmosphere where ideas can be freely shared—and frequently constructively criticized—as they are molded into well-rounded proposals for funding. Teamwork is intrinsic to grant writing, as funding success is often partly based upon the combined strengths and relative potential contribution of each team member. Yet the danger that sometimes befalls imagers is the "hammer and nail" fallacy, that is: "to a man with a hammer everything looks like a nail." Imagers should not worship at the altar of their modality seeking to venerate it above all false gods with equipment-focused proposals. Rather the patient, with a relevant clinical question, should be rightfully placed at the center of the research proposal. The optimum imaging to answer the question posed thus becomes an appropriate secondary consideration dictated by need rather than preference. The sense of detachment from one's favorite modality that needs to be inculcated reaches its logical conclusion when considering comparative effectiveness trials of cardiac imaging. Here, individual team members need to put aside personal prejudices and indeed be willing to see their own modality possibly proven in some way inferior to another in the search for truth. As Oscar Wilde once acerbically remarked, "Anyone can sympathize with the sufferings of a friend but it requires a very fine nature to sympathize with a friend's success." Human nature suggests that such maturity of purpose is the exception rather than the rule in many academic medical centers.

Practical methods for strengthening research in the heart imaging teams include regular research meetings to discuss ideas and present preliminary data; frequent discussion with peers in other areas of cardiology to ascertain the most pressing clinical questions they would like to see answered; pre-review committees prior to grant submission; formal statistical support at no or low cost; favorable imaging rates for generating pilot data; cross-fertilization meetings, for example, with engineers, who rarely have ready access to physicians but may have much to offer; funding to encourage translational working between imagers and basic scientists; and a bottom-up approach to encouraging trainee involvement in meaningful research. Ultimately though, the bedrock for team research is collegiality. Ongoing research should be listed in tabular form and accessible to all team members to avoid duplication of effort and ideas. Teams with members who do not trust or respect each other are unlikely to be productive long term (note that members do not have to *like* each other, but *respect* is fundamentally required at minimum).

Conclusion: The Road Ahead or the Road Less Traveled?

Imaging is in constant evolution, and the heart imaging team faces many challenges as a result. All physicians struggle with keeping up to date, and for a multi-modality cardiac imager, the task seems even more daunting. Imaging costs continue to spiral upward and—on a population basis—the medical radiation dose remains of concern, despite dramatic reductions in radiation exposure achieved at the individual patient level. It would be foolish to imagine that heart imaging teams can solve these problems entirely, but it's reasonable to take ownership of our piece of the problem. This may require us to be more forceful than traditionally has been the case when receiving requests for imaging. Tests that are likely to be of low yield or will not alter management should be gently turned aside and a better strategy discussed with the referring physician. Decision support software may help achieve this at point-of-order in the clinic or on the ward. However, the previous sentence hints at an unacknowledged issue, casual use of the word "order"—should we expect our colleagues to *order a test* or to *request an opinion*? Many would argue that one is shorthand for the other, and yet this is not a meaningless distinction. Rather it cuts to the heart of what an imaging expert should be able to offer. We cannot expect our colleagues to be experts in imaging, nor to understand the clinical variables that may favor one imaging modality over another, and even less to have knowledge of relative waiting list delays in our institutions. Surely the time has come for the heart imaging team to announce "tell us about your patient and tell us what question(s) you wish us to answer—and leave the rest (including choice of test or tests) up to us." This is the road less traveled, but it may be a journey worth undertaking and the road to the right test for the right patient at the right time.

References

1. Leslie A, Jones AJ, Goddard PR. The influence of clinical information on the reporting of CT by radiologists. Br J Radiol. 2000;73(874):1052–5.
2. Mullins ME, Lev MH, Schellingerhout D, Koroshetz WJ, Gonzalez RG. Influence of availability of clinical history on detection of early stroke using unenhanced CT and diffusion-weighted MR imaging. Am J Roentgenol. 2002;179(1):223–8.
3. Wassermann TB, Straus CM. A failure to communicate? Acad Radiol. 2018;25:943.
4. Cohen MD, Curtin S, Lee R. Evaluation of the quality of radiology requisitions for intensive care unit patients. Acad Radiol. 2006;13(2):236–40.
5. Saito JM, Yan Y, Evashwick TW, Warner BW, Tarr PI. Use and accuracy of diagnostic imaging by hospital type in pediatric appendicitis. Pediatrics. 2013;131(1):e37–44.
6. Alkasab TK, Alkasab JR, Abujudeh HH. Effects of a computerized provider order entry system on clinical histories provided in emergency department radiology requisitions. J Am Coll Radiol. 2009;6(3):194–200.
7. Pevnick JM, Herzik AJ, Li X, Chen I, Chithriki M, Jim L, et al. Effect of computerized physician order entry on imaging study indication. J Am Coll Radiol. 2015;12(1):70–4.
8. Ip IK, Schneider LI, Hanson R, Marchello D, Hultman P, Viera M, et al. Adoption and meaningful use of computerized physician order entry with an integrated clinical decision support system for radiology: ten-year analysis in an urban teaching hospital. J Am Coll Radiol. 2012;9(2):129–36.

9. Vartanians VM, Sistrom CL, Weilburg JB, Rosenthal DI, Thrall JH. Increasing the appropriate-ness of outpatient imaging: effects of a barrier to ordering low-yield examinations. Radiology. 2010;255(3):842–9.

10. Min JK, Gilmore A, Budoff MJ, Berman DS, O'Day K. Cost-effectiveness of coronary CT angiography versus myocardial perfusion SPECT for evaluation of patients with chest pain and no known coronary artery disease. Radiology. 2010;254(3):801–8.

11. Sharples L, Hughes V, Crean A, Dyer M, Buxton M, Goldsmith K, et al. Cost-effectiveness of functional cardiac testing in the diagnosis and management of coronary artery disease: a ran-domised controlled trial. The CECaT trial. Health Technol Assess. 2007;11(49):iii–v, ix–115.

12. Thom H, West NE, Hughes V, Dyer M, Buxton M, Sharples LD, et al. Cost-effectiveness of initial stress cardiovascular MR, stress SPECT or stress echocardiography as a gate-keeper test, compared with upfront invasive coronary angiography in the investigation and manage-ment of patients with stable chest pain: mid-term outcomes from the CECaT randomised con-trolled trial. BMJ Open. 2014;4(2):e003419.

13. Pontone G, Andreini D, Guaricci AI, Rota C, Guglielmo M, Mushtaq S, et al. The STRATEGY study (stress cardiac magnetic resonance versus computed tomography coronary angiography for the management of symptomatic revascularized patients): resources and outcomes impact. Circ Cardiovasc Imaging. 2016;9(10):pii:e005171.

14. Sikkens JJ, Beekman DG, Thijs A, Bossuyt PM, Smulders YM. How much overtesting is needed to safely exclude a diagnosis? A different perspective on triage testing using Bayes' theorem. PLoS One. 2016;11(3):e0150891.

15. Doherty JU, Kort S, Mehran R, Schoenhagen P, Soman P. ACC/AATS/AHA/ASE/ASNC/HRS/SCAI/SCCT/SCMR/STS 2017 appropriate use criteria for multimodality imaging in valvular heart disease: a report of the American College of Cardiology appropriate use cri-teria task force, American Association for Thoracic Surgery, American Heart Association, American Society of Echocardiography, American Society of Nuclear Cardiology, Heart Rhythm Society, Society for Cardiovascular Angiography and Interventions, Society of Cardiovascular Computed Tomography, Society for Cardiovascular Magnetic Resonance, and Society of Thoracic Surgeons. J Am Coll Cardiol. 2017;70(13):1647–72.

16. Rybicki FJ, Udelson JE, Peacock WF, Goldhaber SZ, Isselbacher EM, Kazerooni E, et al. 2015 ACR/ACC/AHA/AATS/ACEP/ASNC/NASCI/SAEM/SCCT/SCMR/SCPC/SNMMI/STR/STS appropriate utilization of cardiovascular imaging in emergency department patients with chest pain: a joint document of the American College of Radiology appropriateness criteria committee and the American College of Cardiology appropriate use criteria task force. J Am Coll Cardiol. 2016;67(7):853–79.

17. Patel MR, White RD, Abbara S, Bluemke DA, Herfkens RJ, Picard M, et al. 2013 ACCF/ACR/ASE/ASNC/SCCT/SCMR appropriate utilization of cardiovascular imaging in heart failure: a joint report of the American College of Radiology Appropriateness Criteria Committee and the American College of Cardiology Foundation Appropriate Use Criteria Task Force. J Am Coll Cardiol. 2013;61(21):2207–31.

18. Hendel RC, Lindsay BD, Allen JM, Brindis RG, Patel MR, White L, et al. ACC appropriate use criteria methodology: 2018 update: a report of the American College of Cardiology appro-priate use criteria task force. J Am Coll Cardiol. 2018;71(8):935–48.

19. Cardiac imaging: radiologists move to protect MR and CT turf | diagnostic imaging [Internet]. Available at: http://www.diagnosticimaging.com/nuclear-imaging/cardiac-imaging-radiolo-gists-move-protect-mr-and-ct-turf. Cited 10 Jun 2018.

20. Levin DC, Rao VM. Turf wars in radiology: should it be radiologists or cardiologists who do cardiac imaging? J Am Coll Radiol. 2005;2(9):749–52.

21. Rao VM, Levin DC. Turf wars in radiology: training in diagnostic imaging: how much is enough? J Am Coll Radiol. 2005;2(12):1016–8.

22. Munk PL, Liu DM. Training standards and imaging: will these have any impact on turf wars affecting radiologists? Can Assoc Radiol J. 2010;61(2):66.

23. Levin DC, Rao VM. Turf wars in radiology: updated evidence on the relationship between self-referral and the overutilization of imaging. J Am Coll Radiol. 2008;5(7):806–10.

24. Agarwal R, Levin DC, Parker L, Rao VM. Trends in PET scanner ownership and leasing by nonradiologist physicians. J Am Coll Radiol. 2010;7(3):187–91.
25. Levin DC, Rao VM, Parker L, Frangos AJ, Sunshine JH. Ownership or leasing of CT scanners by nonradiologist physicians: a rapidly growing trend that raises concern about self-referral. J Am Coll Radiol. 2008;5(12):1206–9.
26. Okawa G, Ching K, Qian H, Feng Y. Automatic release of radiology reports via an online patient portal. J Am Coll Radiol. 2017;14(9):1219–21.
27. Wiefels C, Erthal F, deKemp RA, et al. Radionuclide imaging in decision-making for coronary revascularization in stable ischemic heart disease. Curr Cardiovasc Imaging Rep. 2018;11:20.

Implementing Multiple Heart Teams: The University of Ottawa Heart Institute Approach

9

Heather Sherrard and Norvinda Rodger

Introduction

If you are anyone (physician, clinician, administrator) involved in the care of cardiac patients, you have likely heard about "heart teams." Depending on your area of clinical specialization, you may already be participating in a heart team. This concept is gaining traction in today's healthcare environment with a promise of improved collaboration, team decision-making, and patient outcomes. However, changing the structures within which healthcare organizations operate can create significant change and risk. An important consideration for any organization is "should we be implementing heart teams given the limited evidence and lack of clear direction for teams?"

Our organization has adopted heart teams as a new way to approach care, putting in place a formal process to identify and implement teams across the organization. This chapter will outline the processes, challenges, and early learnings of multiple heart team implementations.

The decision to implement numerous teams across a complex organization required a systematic approach. Five key questions were used to guide the decision:

1. What is shifting in the environment to suggest the need for change?
2. Is there good alignment with the organization?
3. Is there evidence to support the decision?
4. What are the risks with this decision?
5. Can any risks be mitigated?

H. Sherrard (✉) · N. Rodger
Department of Clinical Services, University of Ottawa Heart Institute, Ottawa, ON, Canada
e-mail: hsherrard@ottawaheart.ca

© Springer Nature Switzerland AG 2019
T. Mesana (ed.), *Heart Teams for Treatment of Cardiovascular Disease*,
https://doi.org/10.1007/978-3-030-19124-5_9

The Changing Environment

Care of cardiovascular patients has become increasingly complex. Patients are living longer, have multiple chronic conditions, and have an increasing number of treatment options. Cardiovascular care is a technology-rich environment. Each decade's technical advances cause dramatic changes in care options and processes for patient care. Technology now allows for the minimally invasive treatment of valvular conditions in patients who are not eligible for surgery. The evolution of stent products has dramatically shifted the treatment options between interventional cardiology and cardiac surgery. The care and treatment options for arrhythmia patients are still evolving, with new catheter-based procedures and improved surgical options, as well as advancements in anticoagulation therapy.

Numerous clinical trials are reporting results on various combinations of conditions and treatment options. The design rigor associated with randomized clinical trials (RCTs) often makes the application of results increasingly complicated for clinicians who have to operate in the real world across from a patient who might not fit the study parameters. The need for collaboration between multiple specialties in determining and delivering patient treatment options is becoming more and more of a necessity.

A final important consideration is the evolving relationship between patients, families, and healthcare providers. The past decade has seen a significant shift, as many organizations have moved toward models of patient-centered care. This model has more engagement between patients and providers at the individual patient level, but also at the level of program design and development. Because of the complexity of care and the increased engagement of patients, movement toward new models of team-based care is inevitable.

Organizational Alignment

The success of any major change is rooted in its alignment with the organization's vision, mission, and values. Heart teams, as a concept, require the ability to form cross-functional teams, have a culture of working together, and a focus on the patient-care experience. The University of Ottawa Heart Institute (the Institute) has a long history of delivering world-class care. It is an organization with dedicated professionals focused on cardiac patients and a long history of working together. Its actual design puts cardiac surgeons, cardiologists, and cardiac anesthetists together with registered nurses and allied health professionals under one roof and one leadership team. Budgets and resources are shared between all services and are allocated based on patient need. This has created an environment of close collaboration in patient care. The natural experience of patients as they move between the various cardiac services (prevention, rehabilitation, surgery, and cardiology) is mirrored by the structure and processes of the organization. Finally, a key value of the Institute is "our patients come first."

Evidence to Support the Decision

A review of the literature indicates that other organizations are experimenting with heart teams. However, there is no clear definition of a heart team, nor are there many well-established organizational models for implementation of multiple teams which have been tested.

The literature does highlight some effective teams that have been in existence based on a long history of dealing with complex patients. As an example, teams supporting heart failure patients have demonstrated reduced hospitalization, length of stay, and mortality, and improved quality of life [1–3]. More recently the Synergy between Percutaneous Coronary Intervention (PCI) with Taxus and Cardiac Surgery (SYNTAX) trial required a joint review by both a cardiac surgeon and cardiologist on the optimal revascularization strategy. Some agencies now require a "team" approach to transcatheter aortic valve replacement (TAVR) as part of funding based on the review process used by this study.

Given the paucity of evidence in the published literature, the Institute distributed a survey to 38 major cardiac centers across Canada to assess the status of heart teams. More than half (55%) of the organizations responded. Of these, 47.6% did not currently have a heart team in place. Of those that had heart teams, 61% had been in existence for more than 5 years; 38% had been in place for less than 1–2 years. When asked about current roles, 100% of teams were involved in determining treatment options and 92% in patient selection. Developing innovative practices (77%) and fostering clinical research (62%) were the next most common roles.

The Advisory Board recently reported on a survey by the Transcatheter Cardiovascular Therapeutics Symposium (TCT) of 250 clinicians on how they used heart teams. Nearly one-third (29.1%) stated they used them for patient selection; 19.7% used them for all stages of care [4].

Variation in team composition and roles is still evident in the literature. Despite this, there appears to be support for the team concept, given the recent recommendations of several professional associations. The European Society of Cardiology and European Association for Cardiothoracic Surgery Guidelines on Myocardial Revascularization have the heart team concept as a Class 1 recommendation [5]. The ACC/AHA Guidelines for Coronary Artery Bypass Grafting Surgery [6] and the ACC/AHA Guidelines for the management of patients with Valvular Heart Disease [7] also have Class 1 recommendations. The support of this approach by significant professional associations in the absence of traditional evidence suggests the importance of these teams.

Assessment of Risk

The implementation of heart teams has some inherent risks. Depending on the organization, it can be a significant change, with the level of risk related to the degree

of change. The Institute used a risk assessment tool to identify and rank the risks associated with the initiative. The potential risks were a decrease in productivity; increased resistance; multiple major changes occurring at the same time; patient and family perception; provider perception; and unequal adoption (how quick), spread (how many), and proficiency (how well) among the teams.

The risk matrix used to determine the level of risk for the organization and the mitigation strategies which would need to be incorporated into the design and implementation of the team strategy is illustrated in Fig. 9.1.

Impact consequences		Severe	Moderate	Low
Likelihood	Almost certain	Certain risk	High risk 3	Moderate risk
	Likely	High risk	Moderate risk 1,2	Low risk
	Possible	Moderate risk	Low risk 5,6,7,8	Low risk 4

Risk	Risk definition	Mitigation
1. Decrease in productivity	The risk that activities of the team would have a negative impact on workflow (reduce) or the ability to provide services. This could be reductions in procedures; patients days or changes to the cost profile.	Identify metrics based on projects. Consideration to changes in procedure volumes; patient days; length of stay and cost per patient day
2. Resistance to change	The risk that clinicians or support staff would not support the changes and therefore impact the successful implementation of team projects or initiatives	Link to change management resources. For large changes use change tools to assess for readiness and change strategies. Ensure a review of magnitude and impact of change is done for major projects.
3. Multiple changes occurring simultaneously	The risk that multiple heart teams would create several changes simultaneously and the organization or its staff would not be able to adapt quickly enough. This risk could also impact spread and adoption.	To be reviewed by the executive sponsor for timing and impact of implementation. (Heart teams were staged because of a major expansion occurring in 2018)
4. Negative family or patient perception	The risk that recommendations from heart teams would create a cultural shift in the way in which care is delivered to patients which might be negatively perceived by patients or families.	Patient representatives are added to heart teams for input. Patient experience is monitored through patient satisfaction surveys. Consideration can be given to adding specific questions related to a change if needed.
5. Negative provider perception	The risk that recommendations from heart teams would have an impact on current physician workflows which would not be supported by all physicians. This risk is also linked to adoption.	Major changes are tabled at senior management to ensure all members of the leadership team are aware and supportive. Audits of activity and compliance can be done related to specific activities if required.
6. Unequal adoption	The risk that the speed of recommendation adoption would not be similar across the organization. Depending on the recommendation this could have patient safety implications.	Project manager will monitor early adoption as part of the implementation. Workplans and deliverables are tools for monitoring progress
7. Unequal spread	The risk that the roll out of recommendations could be variable among different units in the organization; or that processes or workflows are different on various units.	Project manager works with various units to ensure awareness and consistent adoption
8. Unequal proficiency	The risk that some teams are more capable of developing and implementing heart team activities. This creates additional risks around measuring outcomes and sustainability.	Use of team effectiveness tools and change management resources if there appears to be team capacity issues.

Fig. 9.1 Risk matrix for heart teams

The full review led to a final decision to implement heart teams across the Institute. This strategy has been embedded into the strategic plan and is a metric monitored by the Chief Executive Officer (CEO) and the Board of Governors.

Implementing Heart Teams

In our organization, we used a three-phased approach for implementation (Fig. 9.2): Phase 1, preparing for teams; Phase 2, launching teams; and Phase 3, sustaining teams. Two key enablers—data management and change management—were included in the strategy.

Phase 1: Preparing for Teams

This phase has four key activities: defining a heart team, identifying which teams would be selected, selecting team members, and establishing standard terms of reference.

Defining Teams

The first major challenge was to define a heart team. Team, as it turns out, has diverse meanings. The Oxford dictionary defines "team" as two or more persons working together. The Merriam-Webster dictionary defines team as a "number of persons associated together in work or activity." Wikipedia would conclude a team is a "group of individuals working together to achieve a goal… thus generating performance greater than the sum of the performance of individual members." So, at a minimum a team should comprise two or more people, working toward a goal with an expectation of some improved performance.

More recent definitions reflect the focus of some teams on very specific groups of patients. Nallamothu and Cohen [8] defined a heart team as an integrated, active decision-making between groups of physicians with diverse expertise when therapeutic options exist. Holmes et al. [9] describes heart teams as the use of collective wisdom of various specialties, and identifies and recommends the optimal course of therapy for patients with heart disease.

In today's healthcare environment, the need for cost-effective or value-based care is requiring a shift in the composition and mandate of traditional teams if they are going to be sustainable into the future. In our organization, we have evolved these definitions further. We believe that heart teams are "clusters or groups of multiple clinicians who are focused on the treatment patterns for groups of patients. While they must include consideration for individual patient requirements, they must also look beyond an individual patient and develop

Fig. 9.2 Phases of
implementation

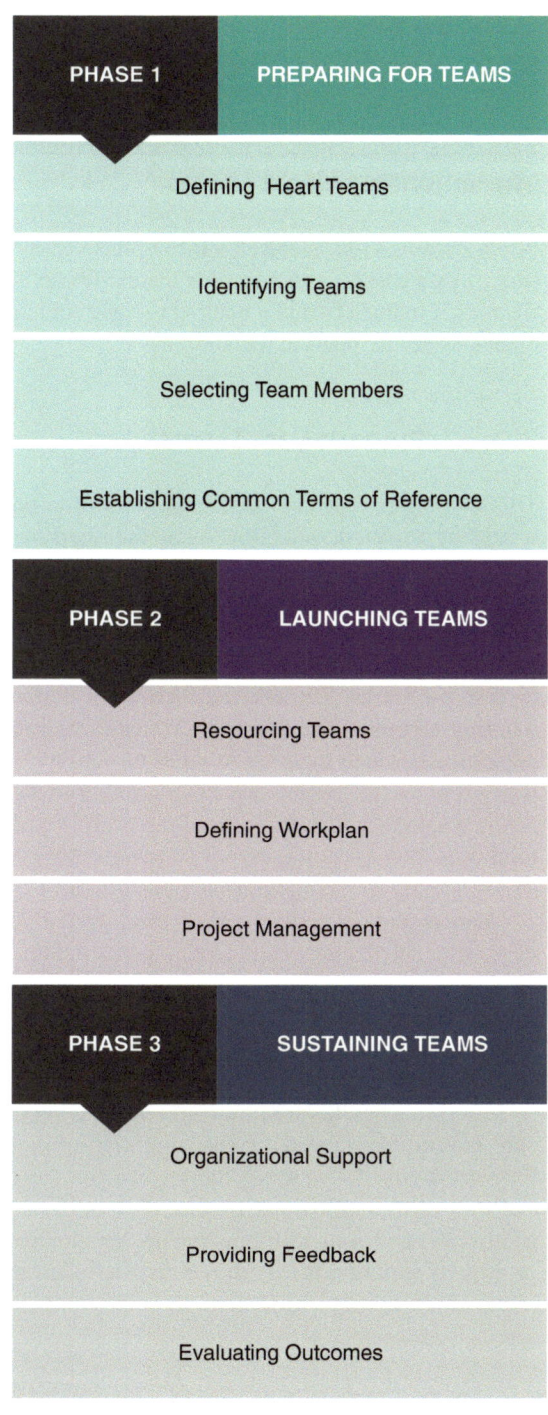

PHASE 1   PREPARING FOR TEAMS

Defining Heart Teams

Identifying Teams

Selecting Team Members

Establishing Common Terms of Reference

PHASE 2   LAUNCHING TEAMS

Resourcing Teams

Defining Workplan

Project Management

PHASE 3   SUSTAINING TEAMS

Organizational Support

Providing Feedback

Evaluating Outcomes

strategies which promote improved outcomes for a broad group of patients. These teams must be structured to deal with the myriad of challenges facing current cardiac patients."

Identifying the Teams

The second step was to identify how many teams the organization would support. Given the full range of teams that could have been possible, the following criteria were used:

- Alignment with the new team definition
- Sufficient critical mass of patients and providers to warrant a team
- Management of complex patient populations
- Early evidence in the literature of a similar team
- Activities of the team could be leveraged to improve care in the community
- Alignment with high-volume, high-complexity, or high-risk activities
- Support a strategic direction of the Institute

Six new heart teams were identified through this process:

1. Coronary artery disease (CAD)
2. Arrhythmia
3. Women's heart health
4. Critical care
5. Cardiac imaging
6. Heart failure

Of note, an existing transcatheter aortic valve replacement (TAVR) team is being expanded to include all structural heart procedures. Heart failure has a long-standing team focused on the specific care and treatment of heart failure. This team will be expanded to include other aspects of a failing heart, such as mechanical circulatory support.

Identifying Team Membership

The membership for each team is defined based on the specific needs of the team (Fig. 9.3). Teams have to include representation from the major medical specialties that care for the patient population. For example, the CAD team has a cardiac surgeon and interventional cardiologist at a minimum. The arrhythmia team has a cardiac surgeon and an electrophysiologist. Additional representation from other medical specialties (imaging, general cardiology, intensive care medicine, anesthesia) are added as appropriate. Teams also include other clinicians such as advanced practice nurses, clinical managers, and allied health staff (physiotherapy, psychology, social work, dieticians). Finally, a patient representative is added to each team to ensure issues important to patients are added to the work plans, as well as to provide feedback from

	Heart Teams					
	Coronary Artery Disease	Arrhythmia	Women's Heart Health	Critical Care	Cardiac Imaging	Heart Failure
Cardiac Surgery					Not Yet Formed	Not Yet Formed
Interventional Cardiology		·	·			
General Cardiology/Heart Failure Specialist	·					
Electrophysiology	·		·	·		
Cardiac Imaging			·	·		
Anesthesia/Critical Care						
Advanced Practice Nurse						
Clinical Manager (RN)						
Psychology	·	·		·		
Physiotherapy	·	·		·		
Technologist		·	·			
Patient				·		
Other	·	·		·		

Fig. 9.3 Comparison of team membership

a patient perspective on team projects. The patient representative is not involved in any specific patient treatment discussions, due to privacy reasons.

The teams vary in size from 11 to 25 members. These teams are slightly larger than usual, but the size allows for some cross coverage and provides additional resources for smaller working groups as needed.

In the first year of startup, medical co-leads are appointed as chairs of the committee, with clearly defined roles and responsibilities. In some cases, the co-leads are department heads, in other situations they are not.

Establishing Common Terms of Reference

The challenge in implementing multiple teams across an organization is three-fold. First, the teams need to remain aligned with the overall corporate strategy. Second, there needs to be clear accountability to allow for a fit within existing (remaining) structures to avoid duplication of effort. Third, the organization needs the ability to monitor and evaluate each of the teams against a common framework. From the onset, the CEO established common terms of reference to guide all teams. Teams have the freedom to pick specific projects or activities, as long as they fit within the terms of reference.

The accountability structure is also embedded within the terms of reference with clear lines of reporting. This is particularly important in the early stages to ensure

appropriate levels of decision-making, and to avoid duplication and confusion within the existing management and university structures. This is key for department heads who may not necessarily be a member of the heart team.

The broad terms of reference are similar for all teams and include specific requirements around innovation, research, and clinical care. The multidisciplinary heart team is responsible for:

1. Developing novel strategies for patient screening; triaging to appropriate treatment and optimal patient follow-up
2. Promoting adherence to best practice with treatment recommendations and services based on best available evidence
3. Developing educational and leadership opportunities for staff who are participating on the team
4. Promoting collaborative clinical research based on the broad disease category of the team
5. Developing a long-term outcome monitoring process with recommendations to senior management
6. Reviewing metrics for the services being provided by the team and making recommendations to senior management as required
7. Identifying opportunities for regional activities in support of the partners that we currently serve

Phase 2: Involves launching the Teams

There are three activities in this phase: resourcing the teams, developing work plans, and establishing project management.

Resourcing

Each of the teams is assessed for support needs based on their work plan. Typically, a team has access to one full-time equivalent to support projects from the work plan. One team used the funds to recruit a nurse, the other an X-ray technologist. These funds are available for the first year and meant to assist teams in launching activities. They are not considered ongoing operating support. Employees of the Institute typically attended meetings and participate in projects as part of their usual work. Meetings and activities are scheduled to accommodate physician attendance, as most physicians in the Institute are fee-for-service. There is no specific remuneration for physician participation on a heart team.

Support is also provided through a project manager funded by the Institute; a vital role in the co-ordination and monitoring of the teams and work plans.

With the launch of the first three teams, the CEO created an innovation fund to provide support for small research projects identified by teams. This is a competitive process, with a detailed submission process and the evaluation of projects headed by the Institute's Chief Scientific Officer. Approved projects receive funds based on progress against the research plan. Research which does not progress has the funding returned to the innovation fund for future redistribution.

Project Management

Early planning has demonstrated the need for project management. The startup of teams, scheduling of meetings, development of work plans, and monitoring of milestones for multiple projects has been essential to the success. The need for this role has become increasingly evident as more heart teams and projects are implemented. As an example, the arrhythmia team has 17 members meeting at two- to three-month intervals. Its first task was to establish a work plan and identify the projects associated with the plan. It has identified five projects including building a triage model, developing a collaborative model for hybrid ablation, designing a program to reduce the incidence of AF in surgical patients, standardizing anticoagulation therapy, and redevelopment and design of educational materials for patients with AF and AF-related procedures. Each of these smaller project teams has its own working group which meets between three and four times to complete their requirements. The resources and support required for each of the working groups vary between 12 and 36 hours per team.

The team has also been successful in acquiring research innovation funds to support three research projects. These projects include improving the outcome with surgical maze, examining the utility of MRI to assess PCI and surgical ablation lesions, and a project to develop a model to assess outcomes on all ablation patients, including an overall measure of quality of life.

The project manager assists with a number of activities beyond a traditional project manager role. These activities can include environmental scans, literature searches, and presentation preparation. The project manager also plays a major role in the monitoring and evaluation as we move through the implementation.

Phase 3: Is Sustaining the Teams

There are three major activities in this phase: ongoing support by the organization, providing feedback, and evaluating outcomes.

Ongoing Support

In order to sustain the heart teams, we have taken several steps to embed them within the organization. The teams were included in the strategic plan and are now supported by other activities being undertaken in the Institute. For example, the heart team concept is integrated into the plans of our research arm.

Another important corporate strategy is to enhance the availability of clinical data for the heart teams. Collaborative, interdisciplinary clinical research with a specific focus on the measurement of long-term outcomes is an expectation of all heart teams.

Historically at the Institute, clinical research databases had been developed by various groups or individuals within the institution, each running on its own unique platform. Data captured routinely as part of day-to-day clinical care is not always automated, and not easily accessible for research purposes. Such a siloed approach was not well aligned with the work being undertaken by the heart teams.

To help support clinical research and the work of heart teams, the CEO led an initiative to create a centralized data platform known as Cardiocore. This is an institution-wide research database which now integrates data elements from procedure- and care-based research modules including percutaneous coronary intervention (PCI), coronary artery bypass graft (CABG), ablation, heart valve, and heart transplant; in addition to critical care modules for both the Coronary Intensive Care Unit (CICU) and Cardiac Surgical Intensive Care Unit (CSICU). The purpose of this initiative is to eliminate duplication, streamline resources and, most importantly, facilitate interdisciplinary research. Standardization of data elements and data definitions was an important first step to ensure integration across modules and to facilitate data sharing. As a member of the Society of Thoracic Surgeons (STS) registry which allows international benchmarking of adult cardiac surgeries, the Institute used the data definitions from this dataset as the standard. All data entered in the STS database is automatically fed into Cardiocore, populating modules that contain the same data fields such as the CABG and CSICU modules; eliminating unnecessary duplication.

To support Cardiocore and the teams that use it, the Institute has consolidated a team of data analysts and data managers. These team members are highly skilled, with a combination of technical, research, and clinical skills, and includes a member with a nursing background and one with a medical degree. This team is responsible for data extraction, data manipulation, data cleaning, and data analysis. It ensures consistency, integrity, and completeness of clinical modules. The Cardiocore team supports the heart teams' data management needs, compiles quality metrics, provides data to support potential and ongoing initiatives, and supports data for publications. This clinical resource will become increasingly important as heart teams link their activities to patient outcomes.

Feedback

Ongoing feedback of team progress is important both at the team and corporate level. Individual heart teams have created a number of smaller working groups to execute specific projects, making it necessary to use a variety of communication tools to ensure all team members are aware of project activities. We use a shared site where all heart teams and members have access to project documents, including progress updates and meeting minutes.

At the corporate level, the executive sponsor provides regular updates of team progress. At the end of the year, each co-chair provides an update of achievements and challenges to the senior management team.

Evaluation of Outcomes

The measurement of outcomes occurs at two levels. The co-leads for each of the teams are responsible for the successful delivery of outcomes for specific projects within the team. These projects are measured against the terms of reference and project deliverables. The project manager provides the team with regular updates on milestones and follows up on activities which are slipping. Each of the team co-leads report back annually to the senior management team to close the accountability loop.

Work plans are used to track activities and support the measurement of outcomes throughout the year. The executive sponsor monitors the broad outcomes of the teams, including project deliverables, resources used, and stability of the team. A sample report template is illustrated in Fig. 9.4.

COMPLEX ARRHYTHMIA HEART TEAM

- Electrophysiologist (EP) (co-chair + 5)
- Cardiac Surgeon (co-chair + 1)
- General Cardiologist
- Anesthetist/Intensivist
- Imaging Cardiologist
- Ambulatory Care Manager
- Triage Coordinator
- Advanced Practice Nurse (APN)
- Unit Manager
- Executive sponsor
- Project manager

*Heart Team members meet 2-3 times per year. Total resourcing commitment estimated at 50+ hours per year. Working Groups time commitment varies by project.

Team Projects

	Triage Model	Collaborative Model for Hybrid Ablation	STOP Afib Program	Standardized Approach to Anti-coagulation	Education – Patients and Providers	Research Project	Long-term Outcome Follow-up
	To develop a virtual clinic model and algorithm to triage AF patients to the appropriate provider to improve access to care and education for patients. To develop AF care map for ED and Family Physicians	To define a collaborative model for Hybrid AF Ablation; a new minimally invasive treatment option (UOHI building expansion will include new Hybrid OR)	To implement an AF preoperative prophylaxis protocol to reduce onset of post-op AF in surgery patients and a postoperative AF treatment algorithm to standardize care	a) To standardize anticoagulation and design a decision algorithm based on patient-preferences b) To identify novel ways of increasing anticoagulation compliance	To identify and design programs and tools for both providers and patients	a) To improve outcomes from concomitant surgical MAZE b) To improve outcomes from surgical stand-alone MAZE procedures c) To examine utility of cardiac MRI to assess PCI and surgical ablation lesions set	To develop a model to assess outcomes of all ablation patients (EP & Surgical) including quality of life

Working Group Participants

	Triage Model	Collaborative Model for Hybrid Ablation	STOP Afib Program	Standardized Approach to Anti-coagulation	Education – Patients and Providers	Research Project	Long-term Outcome Follow-up
	• EP (2) • General Cardiologist (2) • Cardiac Surgeon • APN • Triage Coordinator	• EP (2) • Cardiac Surgeon	• Anesthetist/Intensivist • EP (2) • Cardiac Surgeon • Unit Managers • Educator	• EP (2) • General Cardiologist • Cardiac Surgeon • APN • Ambulatory Care Manager	• EP • Cardiac Surgeon • APN (2) • Triage Coordinator • Unit Manager	• Physician PIs (and research team members)	• EP • Cardiac Surgeon • APN • IT analyst
Meeting Dates							
Status Update							
Completed Deliverables							

Fig. 9.4 Heart team status report template

Challenges and Early Learnings

For organizations wishing to implement multiple heart teams, challenges come at two different levels—at the level of the organization and at the team level. Organizationally, there is a need to determine what kinds of heart teams are needed and appropriately place them inside existing structures, avoiding duplication and confusion in decision-making. The organization also needs to consider the sustainability of the teams and issues such as resourcing and measuring broad outcomes. Finally, depending on the size and number of teams, consideration must be given to managing what may be very diverse teams and activities.

Team Structure

One of the early challenges is in selecting the right members for each team. Initially, individuals want to be involved as it is a new initiative. However, as work begins to progress, some teams experience drift or lack of attendance. This needs to be addressed quickly, as it can have a major negative impact on the team.

Initially, some of our team members were appointed based on a position they held in the Institute. While this may appear desirable, if the individual is a poor participant, our experience would suggest it is better to have a committed team member independent of the leadership role. An alternate approach could be to appoint some members, while allowing others to volunteer based on interest or an application process.

Challenges at the level of team will vary somewhat based on the mandate of the team. A key challenge is the ability to bring busy clinicians together. The scheduling of meetings became an early challenge. It is difficult to determine the need for meetings when the teams are forming; however, physicians needed significant lead time for scheduling because of their clinical and research commitments. We now establish a routine set of meetings in advance to facilitate physician attendance, cancelling them when not needed. We also hold a number of meetings after regular business hours to facilitate attendance.

The work of the heart teams can cause significant changes to current workflows and the need for physician availability. These changes, while beneficial, can be difficult for busy clinicians to accommodate or adapt to. This is particularly true if team activities require the prompt review of cases by physicians from different disciplines. In some cases, the changes may be viewed by some team members as inefficient, which can impact adoption. These difficulties in work flow changes are apparent in CAD teams as they change existing workflows between interventional cardiology and cardiac surgery. Our CAD team, as an example, worked on a process for reviewing patients in the "gray zone" (triple vessel CAD, left main disease, diabetic). Ideally, this should be done at the time of the catheterization; however, this was extremely difficult in practical terms. Rather than abandon the concept, the team has looked at alternatives in terms of a real-time SYNTAX scoring and a surgeon available for review. So rather than the heart team being a deterrent, it becomes an enabler of possible solutions.

The work plans are an important element for successful teams. In year one, teams were able to choose their projects. In subsequent years, we will use a blended model of project selection including those identified by the team and some which may be requested by senior management based on corporate priorities.

Practice Changes

All the teams created practice changes of varying magnitudes. Each change must be properly implemented and nested within the existing organizational structure. For some small changes, this is relatively easy. However, for a significant change, comprehensive change management strategies are needed to ensure good adoption and sustainability of the change. In some instances, we found team members highly engaged in the practice changes, while some of their colleagues remained less committed. Our experience is that considerable time has to be spent on communication with staff who are not directly involved in the discussions to ensure a smooth adoption.

The executive sponsor needs to ensure that the number of changes being proposed by the teams can be properly implemented. In some cases, this may mean staging the implementation. This requires good communication, as it can often be viewed as an unnecessary delay by teams who have worked for some time on a project.

Resourcing

Resourcing of teams can be a challenge. Our current model does not financially reimburse physicians for participation. It does, however, provide project support to minimize the amount of time clinicians have to spend on project activities. The addition of team resources has been valuable to the team success, with each team using their funding in various ways. The CAD team employed a radiology technologist to help with SYNTAX scoring, while the arrhythmia team employed a registered nurse to help with several of the clinical projects.

Measurement of Outcomes

The measuring of outcomes remains a challenge. There is no clear direction in the literature around outcomes. Teams are so diverse that the ability to identify and measure metrics to show the value of teams is still limited. We are beginning with broad outcomes related to the terms of reference, project deliverables, and resourcing. Over the next several years, we envision expanding these to be able to link them to the promise of improved patient outcomes and measures of efficiency and effectiveness.

Conclusion

These heart teams have been developed within a heart institute model whose mandate is cardiac care, research and education. The Institute is an academic center with multidisciplinary cardiac experts all under one roof and a large patient cohort frequently involved in research trials. It has its own management and governance structures and has the ability to allocate funds to specific strategic directions.

There are other organizations in which cardiac care is delivered within the context of a general hospital. Each care-delivery model will have its own strengths/weaknesses when it comes to heart teams. We believe success is rooted in a formal process that identifies teams required on the basis of patient needs.

References

1. Rich MW, Beckham V, Wittenberg C, Leven CL, Freedland KE, Carney RM. A multidisciplinary intervention to prevent the readmission of elderly patients with congestive heart failure. N Engl J Med. 1995;333:1190–5.
2. Stewart S, Marley JE, Horowitz JD. Effects of a multidisciplinary, home-based intervention on planned readmissions and survival among patients with chronic congestive heart failure: a randomised controlled study. Lancet. 1999;354:1077–83.
3. Kasper E, Gerstenblith G, Hefter G. A randomized trial of the efficacy of multidisciplinary care in heart failure outpatients at high risk of hospital readmission. ACC Curr J Rev. 2002;11:57.
4. Titus A. The 'heart team'-defined. In: Advisory Board. Available at: https://www.advisory. com/research/cardiovascular-roundtable/cardiovascular-rounds/2016/05/slsa-heart-team. [Cited 2018 Jul 29].
5. Kolh P, Wijns W. Joint ESC/EACTS guidelines on myocardial revascularization. J Cardiovasc Med. 2011;12:264–7.
6. Hillis LD, Smith PK, Anderson JL, Bittl JA, Bridges CR, Byrne JG, et al. 2011 ACCF/AHA guideline for coronary artery bypass graft surgery: executive summary: a report of the American College of Cardiology Foundation/American Heart Association Task Force on Practice Guidelines. Circulation. 2011;124:2610–42.
7. Nishimura RA, Otto CM, Bonow RO, Carabello BA, Erwin JP, Guyton RA, et al. 2014 AHA/ACC guideline for the management of patients with valvular heart disease: a report of the American College of Cardiology/American Heart Association Task Force on Practice Guidelines. Circulation. 2014;129:e521–643. https://doi.org/10.1161/cir.0000000000000031.
8. Nallamothu BK, Cohen DJ. No "I" in heart team: incentivizing multidisciplinary care in cardiovascular medicine. Circulation. 2012;5:410–3.
9. Holmes DR, Mohr F, Hamm CW, Mack MJ. Venn diagrams in cardiovascular disease: the Heart Team concept. Eur Heart J. 2013;35:66–8.

Multidisciplinary Heart Teams for Cutting-Edge Research

10

Peter P. Liu and Alison M. Hosey

Research Drives Excellence in Science and Clinical Care

Research and innovation are integral to advancement of medical knowledge and resulting improvements in clinical care. It is often said that the "Treatments we enjoy today are fruits of yesterday's research. Tomorrow's cutting-edge care starts with the research today." Canada punches above its weight, as our research output globally is very competitive with research-intensive countries such as the USA and UK in terms of quality and impact [1]—despite a much smaller funding envelope [2] and population. In addition, particularly in the cardiovascular field, the return on investment of research funding has been outstanding—with one estimation of 21% returns annually in perpetuity [3].

Medical knowledge and innovation today advance so quickly that we often forget that aseptic surgery was first performed only 100 years ago and that coronary artery bypass surgery, taken for granted today, was first described by Favaloro 50 years ago [4]. Moreover, the first randomized clinical trial of drug-eluting stent was published in 2002 [5], while trans-aortic valvular replacement (TAVR) was first described in 2006 [6], and the first trial comparing TAVR with surgery was as recently as 2017 [7].

Advancements in technology, communication networks, global collaboration, and increased investments in research are accelerating at an unprecedented pace. While this progress is excellent for patients and cardiovascular care, it also mandates academic institutions and research teams to organize research and innovation

P. P. Liu (✉)
University of Ottawa Heart Institute, Departments of Medicine/Cellular and Molecular Medicine, Ottawa, ON, Canada
e-mail: pliu@ottawaheart.ca; peter.liu@utoronto.ca

A. M. Hosey
University of Ottawa Heart Institute, Research Services, Ottawa, ON, Canada

© Springer Nature Switzerland AG 2019
T. Mesana (ed.), *Heart Teams for Treatment of Cardiovascular Disease*,
https://doi.org/10.1007/978-3-030-19124-5_10

endeavors very deliberately, or they risk being left behind. While busy clinician and health provider teams try to address their clinical patient challenges, the solution is often within the research occurring all around, but with barriers to accessibility for the clinician. Specific advancements in digital health technology and information sharing are breaking down those barriers—rewriting the rules of interface between research and clinical care—and creating new opportunities for collaboration.

Indeed, whether we are dealing with a patient with acute myocardial infarction, heart failure, or arrhythmias, we rely primarily on clinical guidelines and on the latest information gleaned from clinical trial results, cohort studies, meta-analyses, and other information derived from research to determine the path forward.

It is the aggregate of research evidence that inform the clinical guidelines, and in turn this ultimately derives the performance metrics and quality indicators used to monitor outcomes of our clinical care. These evidence-based performance metrics in turn calibrate the reimbursement for care, and the infrastructure support enabling the best care to our patients.

At the same time, it is fundamental research that enhances our understanding of disease mechanisms, and opens the door to new diagnostic and therapeutic innovations. It is only through fundamental science that we learned the roles of inflammation in atherosclerosis, remodeling in heart failure, and re-entry in cardiac arrhythmias. The fundamental understanding of immune regulation led to new immune checkpoint therapies in cancer that are transforming treatment and changing lives. This particular discovery by Professors James Allison and Tasuku Honjo was awarded the 2018 Nobel Prizes in Medicine, a testament to the power of fundamental research. The recent advances in small interfering RNA (siRNA) as therapies for cholesterol-lowering through PCSK9 inhibition [8], or blocking amyloid formation for regression of neuropathy or restrictive heart failure [9], are all derived from fundamental research discoveries. Through translation of discoveries, and the addition of innovative tools for disease treatment (and indeed prevention), advances such as these promise to reshape the future of medicine and the treatment of cardiovascular disorders.

Research Today Requires a Multidisciplinary Team Effort

Research advances today require a team of experts to solve a problem in an integrated fashion. The classic model of the single investigator working with a student making an earth-shattering discovery has become the stuff of legend. Modern research is incredibly complex (in concept and technology), making fundamental high-impact observation no longer readily within the reach of a single investigator. Even if such an observation did occur, it would be impossible to translate to meaningful impact on humans without a team of experts from multiple disciplines.

For example, gaining a complete understanding of the fundamental biological pathways underpinning complex diseases such as heart failure or atherosclerosis requires the convergence of molecular and cellular biology, genetics, systems biology, animal models, human materials, and bioinformatics. Indeed, one would need

to work with top experts to bring together diverse technology, scientific insights, convergence of multiple observations, and datasets, to derive new fundamental principles. For example, the understanding of stem cell biology, the ability to reprogram somatic cells into mature cell lineage using the Yamanaka factors, and then programming forward into differentiated brain or heart cells to assembly microorgans, or organoids, require a significant repertoire of expertise and technologies with stringent controls and robust protocols.

Similarly, to conduct a diagnostic or therapeutic evaluation in patients, modern clinical trials require collaborations among global leading centers to share expertise and to recruit qualified patients effectively. Many clinical trials require hundreds of investigators and their teams, including nurses, technicians, and laboratory personnel, to collect relevant and robust data to answer a major question. It is no longer possible for a single clinician, making bedside observations, to hope to influence the field (as in the early days of Sir William Osler).

To maximize impact for medical discovery, fundamental innovations need to be applied at the bedside. To do translational science requires even more complex collaboration. The teams will need to include fundamental research members from multiple disciplines (e.g., chemists for drug discovery), clinical research experts, and methodologists, with additional inputs from patients, end-users, and regulatory authorities, to ensure the transition of knowledge from those who discovered it to those who knows how to use it, and everyone in between who can enable this process to succeed and make a clinical impact. The same is true for clinician observations that need to be communicated back to fundamental scientists as problems requiring discovery-based solutions or innovations to meet the gap in clinical care.

Developing a Research Strategy to Meet Today's Needs in Clinical Care: The ORACLE Example

To promote successful team research to address today's complexities, while focused on maximizing impact, a deliberate and carefully developed research strategy is critical. The strategy needs to be able to engage the diverse community of researchers in different disciplines, while changing the culture from individual siloed programs to multidisciplinary team problem-solving. The strategy will also need to allow prioritization and efficient use of resources, leverage partnerships, and promote a robust training environment. To maximize success, one must solicit broad input, with multilayered participation to garner the best ideas, to ensure ownership and adoption. Then, a clear strategy and implementation plan are critical, to perfect the delicate dance between stakeholder buy-in and meaningful and specific priorities of focus.

To accomplish this at the University of Ottawa Heart Institute, we consulted broadly to develop a new research strategic plan for the entire Ottawa-based cardiovascular community. The Ottawa Region for Advanced Cardiovascular Research Excellence, or the ORACLE, strategy was developed following these principles. We

consulted extensively with leadership teams, junior and senior researchers, trainees, partners, stakeholders, and patients. We solicited the best ideas to deliver on our goals of scientific excellence by solving big problems together.

We started out with a fact-finding mission and process, seeking broad engagement. This was followed by working group discussions focusing on specific challenges or tasks, leading up to broad prioritization. By distilling the wisdom and recommendations of the various multidisciplinary teams, we developed, through collaboration, an integrated blueprint to go forward.

One of the key concepts of the ORACLE research plan is the formation of solution-seeking Innovation Hubs, comprised of multidisciplinary investigators and clinicians. The Hubs are focused on some of the most important challenges facing cardiovascular medicine. Examples of these challenges include heart failure with preserved ejection fraction, improved classification of atrial fibrillation, and predicting when an atherosclerotic plaque will rupture. The Hubs are designed to prioritize the important problems, and to break down challenges into discrete solvable projects [7] where multidisciplinary teams can deploy their expertise and unique resources to fast-track solutions.

The multidisciplinary members for each Hub may consist of fundamental biologists, engineers, chemists, computational specialists, cardiologists, epidemiologists, cardiovascular surgeons, psychologists, and physiologists. Some members (such as our Institute Heart Team cardiologists or surgeons) highlight a key problem to the group using case studies or other means; others bring important points of view to the problem-solving exercise, and together the interrelated multidisciplinary team works in a coordinated fashion to design and implement studies to address the problem. The solution to the problem may come from large-scale analysis of linked existing data sources; re-analysis of existing basic science systems biology data; mining our biobank of blood and tissue samples, or clinical trial or large epidemiological databases, to evaluate potential hypotheses, but also to identify critical knowledge gaps. They may also be tested in novel cellular, animal, or human cell models. This may lead to testing directly in detailed patient studies to unravel pathophysiology, or critically evaluate novel diagnostic or therapeutic opportunities. Each of these interdisciplinary projects contributes to the overall cycle of discovery, validation, and knowledge translation (Fig. 10.1). Learning gained from one Hub can sometimes also help to unlock solutions in another Hub, and many investigators move from Hub to Hub to participate in the most exciting problems to solve.

Operationalizing the Hub Concept

Because of the diverse interests in our large clinical and research community, the number of topics that Hubs can investigate is numerous. However, in order for Hubs to function effectively, they must be focused, addressing major problems with high potential impact, and endowed with critical mass of expertise. To determine the most effective number of Hubs, we aggregated the proposed topics, developed a simplified short list, and prioritized based on factors such as burden of disease, size of the knowledge gap, and available local expertise from diverse disciplines that can find solutions expeditiously.

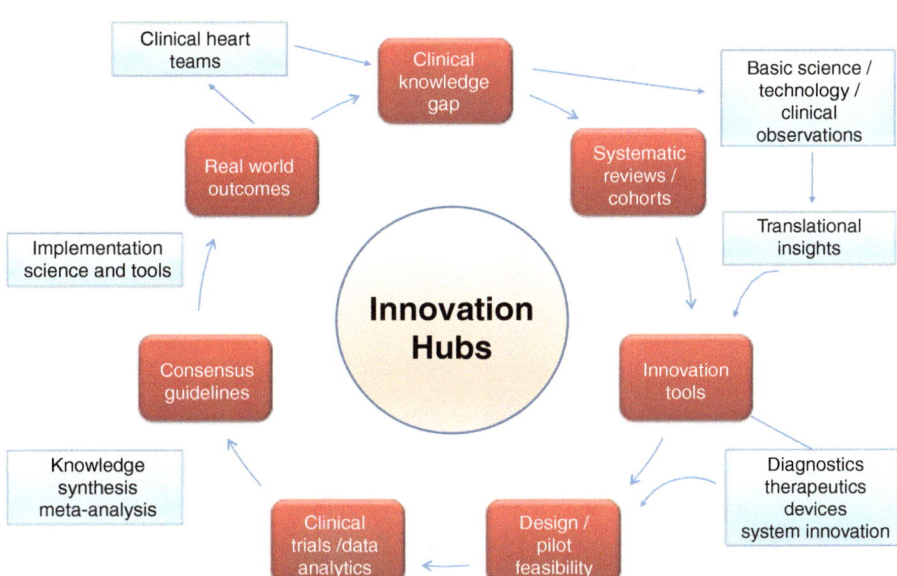

Fig. 10.1 The Innovation Hub Cycle starts out by identifying clinical knowledge gaps and then addressing these gaps through systematic reviews and basic science models and, in turn, discoveries. The resulting insights and innovative tools can then be piloted and properly tested in formalized clinical trials in patient cohorts. The results will inform the evidence for clinical guidelines. New gaps in knowledge can be identified again, and the cycle moves forward in a continuous manner

Initially, more than 20 potential topics were identified. However, through research, data analysis, discussions, and deliberations, we focused on a handful of short-listed topics and landed on five topics. Nevertheless, these Hub topics are designed to evolve in focus and priorities over time as the knowledge and practice advance (Fig. 10.2).

Most of these Hub topics are also major clinical disease categories. For example, Hub foci have included heart failure, atherosclerosis, cardiometabolic diseases, valvular heart diseases, and cardiac arrhythmias. Each Hub attracts expertise from basic science to clinical trials to epidemiology, as well as investigators from disciplines outside of medicine and biology to fast-track solutions. Each Hub has elected co-leaders and organized brainstorming and project update sessions according to its own Hub dynamics. Hubs are provided with some facilitation support from Research Services staff members which serves to keep busy people on track and on top of their responsibilities to the Hub. Each Hub is assigned methodological support, to ensure excellence in study design, as well as a staff or researcher representative from our Institute's Canadian Women's Heart Health Centre to ensure projects are considering sex and gender aspects. Small envelopes of seed funding are released periodically, which are competed for through a rigorous external peer review. The best pilot projects are funded and weighted highest toward the scientific excellence of the proposal and feasibility for maximum impact.

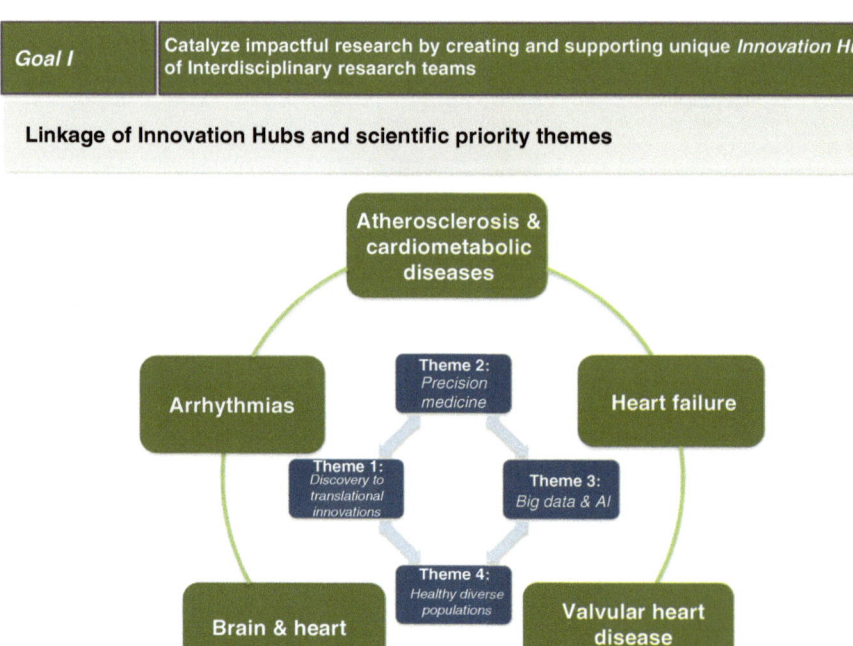

| Goal I | Catalyze impactful research by creating and supporting unique *Innovation Hubs* of Interdisciplinary resaarch teams |

Linkage of Innovation Hubs and scientific priority themes

Fig. 10.2 The innovation hubs are also seamlessly linked to the scientific priorities that cross-cut all hubs of multidisciplinary teams. The themes include (1) effective translation; (2) precision medicine; (3) big data and artificial intelligence tools; and (4) diverse populations

For example, the current Hub on arrhythmias is focused on the problem of atrial fibrillation as the primary priority, with a subconcentration of ventricular arrhythmias leading to sudden death. The Hub projects include the identification of subtypes of atrial fibrillation using big data and AI algorithms. In parallel, there are projects examining various underlying pathophysiology of atrial arrhythmias, using reprogrammed human myocytes in culture, or gene-edited mouse models. There are also projects developing and validating novel biomarkers to facilitate the identification of subtypes of atrial fibrillation. These studies are supported by a robust biobanking effort, so that patient blood and tissue samples are readily available. There are clinical trial teams investigating means of detecting atrial fibrillation early and whether optimizing anticoagulation to prevent stroke is worthwhile in this situation. Patients particularly are enthusiastic on projects aimed to explore psychosocial and behavioral insights for patients with atrial arrhythmias. A project on the best method of exercise and atrial fibrillation is one study coming out of these discussions with patients. The contributions of sympathetic activation and the crosstalk between brain and heart circuits and rhythms are also completely novel areas of scientific exploration being undertaken by this Hub.

Patient Participation in Hub Activities

As the shared aim of clinical care and multidisciplinary research is to improve the lives of our patients, we have actively solicited patients who are part of our patient alumni organization at the Institute, to act as patient partners in Hub research activities (Fig. 10.3). Currently, we have patients with relevant lived experience participating in the Hub activities. Many of these patients have the relevant condition, or have recovered from it. Some are spouses, family members, or caregivers of former or current patients. The patient partners have been invaluable in relating their own personal experiences in the disease encounter, helping to bring to focus the priorities from their point of view, and what the research results will mean for their lives. Their stories have been heartfelt and enlightening. Health researchers don't always understand the emotion or anxiety impact of a disease condition, and what it means to be so short of breath or not knowing when the heart is going to race again, or when the patient may risk passing out. Some of these stresses can lead to depression and difficulties in coping. Our patient partners are fully engaged and anxious to find solutions to their own personal predicaments, or simply to help others to find better life and outcome.

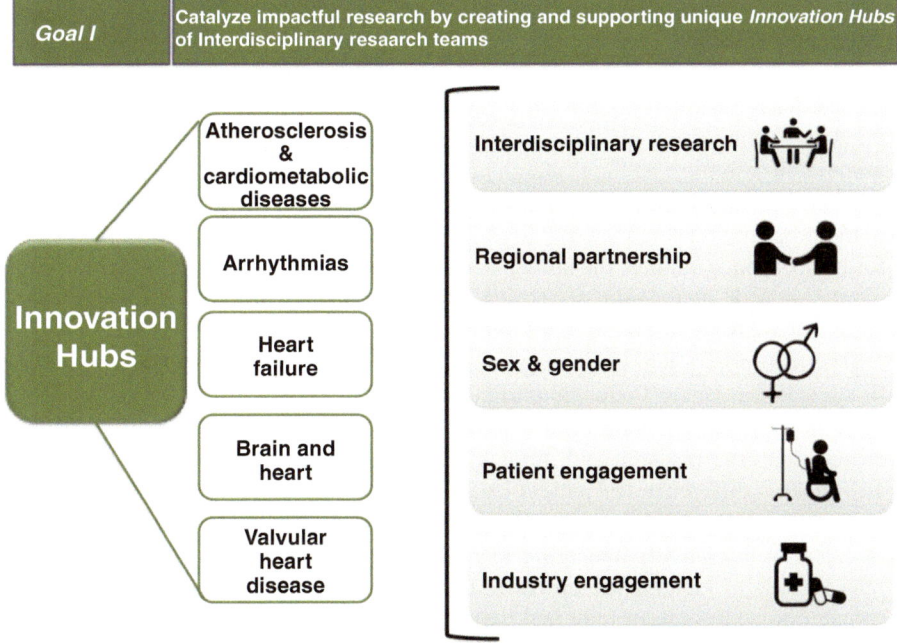

Fig. 10.3 All of the activities of the Innovation Hubs also incorporate key domains of interactions, including interdisciplinary research, regional partnerships, sex and gender considerations, patient engagement, and industry/commercialization, in order to maximize success and impact

Our patient partners participate in a wide variety of Hub activities, from research strategic planning exercises to identifying domains of research that investigators may miss, to devising patient-relevant outcomes. Patients are also excellent participants in individual research projects, where they can help to facilitate the conduct of the trials, or to engage other patients to improve recruitment, or enhance protocol adherence. Patients act as reviewers for our seed-funding competitions, as a complement to the scientific review. They provide excellent review and feedback to the teams, and have tipped the balance of one project getting funding over another, based on their feedback on the projects' relevance to or engagement of patients.

Patients are also instrumental in knowledge translation, and the application of research results. The information and the new data coming through research are much embraced by the patients, particularly if they have been involved in the research itself. The patients become the best ambassadors to propagate the new information to other patients, and help to work with media with their personal stories, to broaden the impact of the research. Patients are also adept in helping to develop tools to apply the findings at the bedside or at home, or tools to monitor the responses to treatments, and/or patient adherence to treatments.

Integrated Knowledge Translation with the Hubs

Research discoveries remain theoretical, until the new information can be translated into innovative tools, guidelines, or benefits that are tangible or can impact on knowledge or patient care. In order for the research activities to have impact, knowledge translation planning and the integration are included as part of the Hub innovation activities. At the research proposal stage, pilot grant application, or peer-reviewed agency submission, tailored approaches to knowledge translation relevant to the proposed research are already included as part of the research protocol. Even for basic science studies, the ability to translate the new findings into specific tools, biomarkers, or therapeutic strategies that can be used by clinical researchers or other scientists should be thought out proactively.

The incorporation of knowledge users into the various Hubs, including clinicians in the relevant Heart Teams, is particularly important to maximize impact. In this way, the clinical knowledge gaps can be addressed by the knowledge users working closely with the research and innovation teams, to develop specific solutions that will make a difference for patient care and outcomes. This incorporation of clinicians in the Hub activities also has the positive effect of getting clinicians involved in research. Frequently, engaging in research can be a barrier for clinicians, who may be able to identify the problem, but do not know where to start to undertake research to address it, or may feel they do not have the time to find experts to help. In the Hub setting, clinicians can input their problem into the wheel of expertise, and then work with the experts to address it. This is empowering for clinicians, and clinicians can, over time, evolve into active investigators.

Other key members of the knowledge translation enablers for the Hubs include technology transfer experts and health system and health policy experts, as well as patients and their families. They all play a key role to complement the multidisciplinary Hub expertise.

Accountability and Feedback of Research Hub Teams

To ensure that the Hubs are able to deliver on solutions in a timely manner, we have set up milestones for each Hub, including specific process indicators, such as the number of meetings or working group brainstorming sessions, and the number of integrated problems identified to be solved. More importantly, we track closely how many of these ideas for pilot projects turn into full protocols, submitted for competitive funding locally or nationally with acquired preliminary data, and how many are funded. With peer-reviewed funding, the teams are well on their way to acquire definitive data to reach conclusions that can influence scientific thinking or patient care at the bedside.

To achieve this, the Hubs meet regularly, e.g., every 2–3 months, depending on the phase of Hub development, to review progress and determine course of action. The Hubs need to set up a specific work plan with milestones and metrics to be eligible for funding opportunities.

Not all the Hubs progress at the same rate. Some Hubs are extremely vibrant, with the members regularly coming up with exciting cutting-edge ideas. Many of these are extremely successful in attracting pilot funding. They rapidly gather proof-of-concept data using existing infrastructure and become, in a short time, well poised to compete for—very often successfully—major peer-reviewed funding. This creates an exciting positive-feedback environment to attract the best trainees, other investigators, and international partners.

On the other hand, some of the Hubs struggle to generate momentum. Some of the difficulty is due to the lack of resources with a brand new Hub. In other cases, there may be a lack of effective leadership. There may be lack of motivation if pilot projects do not get funded through our internal competitions, as adjudication is based on excellence in science rather than spreading the funds per Hub. These Hubs will garner extra attention from the Chief Scientific Officer and the Research Services support team. The administration will engage the Hub team and external scientific advisors to get the Hub back on track, with celebration of even small wins. Ultimately, most of the Hubs become productive in time, and become nexus of innovation, and also foster careers, training opportunities, and excellent productivity. Once successful, the Hubs become perpetual self-organizing units of discovery and knowledge translation.

Conclusion

Research is a dynamic and constantly evolving process, improving our understanding of disease processes, developing better tools of care, and monitoring patient outcomes. With the emergence of new molecular targets, drug delivery methods, smart devices, and improved process of care, the future is exciting, but will require more exacting research. With improved tools including multi-modality high-resolution imaging, big data, and physiological event monitoring, artificial intelligence analytic algorithms, and efficient and practical clinical trial methodology, research will accelerate in pace and impact. The research teams of the future will need to be more nimble, efficient, productive, and outcome-oriented, accelerating excellence in care beyond imagination today.

References

1. Nguyen HV, de Oliveira C, Wijeysundera HC, Wong WW, Woo G, Grootendorst P, et al. Canada's contribution to global research in cardiovascular diseases. Can J Cardiol. 2013;29:742–6.
2. de Oliveira C, Nguyen VH, Wijeysundera HC, Wong WW, Woo G, Liu PP, et al. How much are we spending? The estimation of research expenditures on cardiovascular disease in Canada. BMC Health Serv Res. 2012;12:281.
3. de Oliveira C, Nguyen HV, Wijeysundera HC, Wong WW, Woo G, Grootendorst P, et al. Estimating the payoffs from cardiovascular disease research in Canada: an economic analysis. CMAJ Open. 2013;1:E83–90.
4. Favaloro RG. Saphenous vein autograft replacement of severe segmental coronary artery occlusion: operative technique. Ann Thorac Surg. 1968;5:334–9.
5. Morice MC, Serruys PW, Sousa JE, Fajadet J, Ban Hayashi E, Perin M, et al. A randomized comparison of a sirolimus-eluting stent with a standard stent for coronary revascularization. N Engl J Med. 2002;346:1773–80.
6. Webb JG, Chandavimol M, Thompson CR, Ricci DR, Carere RG, Munt BI, et al. Percutaneous aortic valve implantation retrograde from the femoral artery. Circulation. 2006;113:842–50.
7. Smith CR, Leon MB, Mack MJ, Miller DC, Moses JW, Svensson LG, et al. Transcatheter versus surgical aortic-valve replacement in high-risk patients. N Engl J Med. 2011;364:2187–98.
8. Fitzgerald K, White S, Borodovsky A, Bettencourt BR, Strahs A, Clausen V, et al. A highly durable RNAi therapeutic inhibitor of PCSK9. N Engl J Med. 2017;376:41–51.
9. Suhr OB, Coelho T, Buades J, Pouget J, Conceicao I, Berk J, et al. Efficacy and safety of patisiran for familial amyloidotic polyneuropathy: a phase II multi-dose study. Orphanet J Rare Dis. 2015;10:109.

Index

© Springer Nature Switzerland AG 2019

T. Mesana (ed.), *Heart Teams for Treatment of Cardiovascular Disease*,
https://doi.org/10.1007/978-3-030-19124-5